YOUR RIGHTS

to money benefits 2010/2011

Contributors to this book: Sally West, Alban Hawksworth, Sheelagh Donovan, Anna Nalecz, Michael Roche and Jenny Rhys

Age UK thanks the Department for Work and Pensions (DWP) for its comments on the text.

Published by Age UK,
207-221 Pentonville Road, London N1 9UZ

© 2010 Age UK

Thirty-eighth Edition

Editor: Sarah Price
Production: Keith Hawkins

A catalogue record for this book is available from the British Library.

ISBN: 978-0-86242-455-8

We hope that this publication has been useful to you; if so we would very much like to hear from you. Alternatively, if you feel that we could add or change anything, then please write and tell us.

Typeset by: Design and Media Solutions, Maidstone, Kent

Printed in Great Britain by: Colibi Press Ltd, London

Age UK is the new force combining Age Concern and Help the Aged. With almost 120 years of combined history to draw on, we are bringing together our talents, services and solutions to do more to enrich the lives of people in later life.

FSC
Mixed Sources
Product group from well-managed forests and other controlled sources
Cert no. SA-COC-001853
www.fsc.org
© 1996 Forest Stewardship Council

Contents

Introduction

Your Rights to Money Benefits provides information about the main financial benefits and entitlements available for older people. Most of the information applies to those over the qualifying age for Pension Credit, which is rising from 60 to 65 between April 2010 and April 2020, in line with women's State Pension age. The benefit rates given generally apply from the week beginning 12 April 2010. The book is divided into five parts. The first section gives details about pensions and retirement, and the second section is about financial help for those on low incomes. The third part covers benefits and financial support for disabled people and their carers, including the system of help towards paying for care, while the fourth gives information about other types of financial help.

Many of the subjects covered in *Your Rights to Money Benefits* can be complicated, and the book aims to explain them as simply as possible. However, it cannot cover all situations and circumstances. If you need more information, the fifth section gives details about obtaining relevant leaflets from the Department for Work and Pensions (DWP) and Age UK information and about contacting other local and national sources of help. There is also an index and on pages 212–213 a summary of the main benefit rates.

The State pensions and benefits described in this book are delivered through DWP agencies: The Pension, Disability and Carers Service (PDCS) and Jobcentre Plus. Two agencies, The Pension Service and the Disability and Carers Service, have merged to form the PDCS, although for the time being they continue to use their separate names –

which is how they are described in this book. There is more information about this and how to contact the relevant office on pages 198–201. Older people will mainly deal with The Pension Service – either through one of the regional pension centres or the local Pension Service.

Please note that although some older people have young families, benefits for children are not covered in this book. People with dependent children or who are under the qualifying age for Pension Credit should contact a local advice agency or Jobcentre Plus office for information about benefit entitlements.

Where you live in the United Kingdom

All the information covered in *Your Rights to Money Benefits* applies to people living in England. It also applies to Scotland and Wales except where differences are pointed out in the text. Although there is a separate social security system in Northern Ireland, the social security benefits available are generally the same. However, there may be some differences in the sources of financial help discussed in Part 4 'Other Benefits and Financial Support' and local and national sources of further information will also be different.

> *FOR MORE INFORMATION relating to older people living in Scotland, contact the Scottish Helpline for Older People (SHOP) on 0845 125 973; for Wales call Age UK Advice on 0800 169 65 65; for Northern Ireland call 0808 808 7575. Address details can be found on page 224.*

If you are living in the UK but subject to immigration control, your benefit position may be affected. This book does not provide information about immigration status, so contact a local advice agency if you need further details.

Living abroad

Many of the benefits covered in this book will not apply to you if you are living abroad permanently, or they may stop during a temporary stay abroad. In some cases there are special rules for people who live in the European Economic Area (EEA). The EEA is made up of all the European Union countries plus Iceland, Liechtenstein and Norway. The same rules also apply to Switzerland, even though it is not a member of the EEA. Gibraltar is treated as a separate state for social security purposes.

As this book does not give full details about the benefit position for people living abroad, for more information contact your pension centre (if you are currently in this country) or the International Pension Centre, The Pension Service, Tyneview Park, Whitley Road, Benton, Newcastle upon Tyne NE98 1BA, Tel: 0191 218 7777; this is the part of the DWP that deals with pensions and benefits paid abroad.

Pensions

This part of *Your Rights to Money Benefits* contains information about the State Pension, including changes to the rules that were introduced on 6 April 2010. There is also a section that describes what is available to people before and after State Pension age plus details about the Christmas Bonus (paid to people receiving a State Pension or certain other benefits); the procedure for appealing against a social security decision; and occupational and personal pensions.

STATE PENSIONS

The State Pension is paid to people who have reached State Pension age (see below), fulfil the National Insurance (NI) contribution conditions and have made a claim. The amount you get is not affected by your income and savings but it is taxable.

Some major changes to State Pensions were introduced on 6 April 2010. They include the start of a move to gradually increase State Pension age for women from 60 to 65 by April 2020. There are also other changes that will apply to people who reach State Pension age on or after 6 April 2010. In this book we give information about the new rules and the position for people who reached State Pension age before 6 April 2010.

You can claim and get your State Pension even if you are still working past State Pension age. Alternatively, you can choose not to claim your State Pension at State Pension age and instead get extra State Pension or a one-off taxable lump-sum payment at a later date.

Your State Pension may consist of a Basic State Pension plus an Additional State Pension (based on your national insurance contributions record after April 1978) and a Graduated Retirement Benefit (based on your NI contributions record between April 1961 and April 1975). You will get an extra 25p each week when you reach the age of 80. These different parts of the State Pension are explained below. Whether you are entitled to a State Pension or not, you may be able to claim other benefits, such as Pension Credit, Housing Benefit and Council Tax Benefit, which depend on your income and savings.

FOR MORE INFORMATION, see State Pensions – Your Guide, *which is available on the Direct Gov website (www.direct.gov.uk).*

State Pension age

Before 6 April 2010 State Pension age was 65 for men and 60 for women born on or before 5 April 1950. From 6 April 2010 women's State Pension age is being increased, so by 2020 it will be 65 for both men and women. If you are a woman and were born on or after 6 April 1950 and on or before 5 April 1955 your State Pension age will be between 60 years and 1 month and 64 years and 11 months, depending on your date of birth. Every two months over this period State Pension age for women will rise by one month – the precise age at which you are entitled to get your State Pension will depend on your date of birth. (For more information, see the State Pension age calculator on the Direct Gov website, pensions.direct.gov.uk/en/state-pension-age-calculator/home.asp, or ring the State Pension Forecasting Team on 0845 300 0168).

Other benefits, which before 6 April 2010 were paid from the age of 60, may also now be linked to women's State Pension age. The relevant sections of this book will give information about the age at which people become entitled to the different payments.

As a result of changes introduced by *The Pensions Act 2007*, State Pension age will gradually increase from 65 to 68 for both men and women in three stages between 2024 and 2046. This will affect anyone born after 5 April 1959. However, the Government plans to review the date at which the State Pension age starts to rise to 66.

Couples

From 6 April 2010 State Pension provisions are being equalised so they will apply to husbands and wives and people in registered civil partnerships. In the past some pension rights such as the married woman's pension did not apply to husbands and civil partners. Pension changes are generally not retrospective, which means that if your wife or civil partner was born before 6 April 1950 (so reached State Pension age before 6 May 2010, in the case of a woman, or 6 April 2015, in the case of a man) these new rules will not apply to you.

BASIC STATE PENSION

The Basic State Pension is paid at the same rate to everyone who has fulfilled the NI contribution conditions. The full weekly rates are:

Single person	£97.65
Wife on husband's NI contributions record	£58.50
Married couple on husband's NI contributions record	£156.15
Couple *(if both have full NI contributions records)*	£195.30

You may hear the terms 'Category A' and 'Category B' State Pensions. Category A State Pensions are generally based on an individual's own NI contributions record, while Category B State Pensions are based on a spouse or civil partner's record – for example, the State Pension paid to married women or a widow/er or bereaved civil partner. Both types of State Pension consist of a basic and/or Additional State Pension.

Who qualifies?

You will get the full Basic State Pension if you have paid, been treated as having paid or been credited with NI contributions at the appropriate rate for enough qualifying years in your working life, or if any gaps in your record are covered by credited NI contributions or Home Responsibilities Protection (HRP), as explained later. If you do not have sufficient qualifying years for the full Basic State Pension, you may get a reduced Basic State Pension. More information about the NI contribution conditions is given on pages 11–13. They changed on 6 April 2010 and the rules that apply to you will depend on whether or not you reached State Pension age on or after that date.

Normally you need to have satisfied the NI contribution conditions in your own right. However, married women, divorcees, widowed people and those whose civil partnership has ended through bereavement or dissolution may be able to claim a State Pension on their spouse/partner's or former or ex spouse/partner's NI contributions record, as explained in the following pages.

The Category B State Pension for married women

If you are a married woman and you are not entitled to a Basic State Pension based on your own NI contribution record, or you are entitled to a Basic State Pension of less than £58.50 a week, you may be able to get a Basic State Pension based on your husband's NI contributions once he reaches State Pension age. If you are not entitled to a Basic State Pension you can claim a Category B State Pension of £58.50 a week if your husband has a full NI contribution record. This is sometimes referred to as the 'married woman's pension'. If your Basic State Pension is less than £58.50 a week it can be made up to that amount. However, the State Pension 'overlaps' with certain other benefits so, for example, if you were receiving Carer's Allowance this would stop if you started to claim a State Pension that was worth more than the allowance.

If you are already receiving a State Pension on your own NI contributions record and your husband claims his State Pension, The Pension Service will normally pay you any Category B State Pension that you are entitled to so you will not need to make a new claim. You will still need to make a claim if you are not already getting your State Pension at the time your husband reaches State Pension age or if your husband decides to put off claiming his State Pension. Until 6 April 2010 your husband had to be getting his State Pension before you could make a claim but now it is possible to do this even if he is putting off claiming his State Pension. See pages 28–34 for more about putting off claiming the State Pension. If he is putting off claiming his State Pension you should contact The Pension Service to claim the Category B pension even if you are already getting some State Pension based on your own contributions, as it will not be awarded automatically.

On top of any Basic State Pension you get, you may also be entitled to Graduated Retirement Benefit and/or Additional State Pension based on any NI contributions you have made, as explained on pages 22–27 and 28.

Sometimes married women who have paid NI contributions in the past but who are not working when they reach State Pension age do not realise that they may be entitled to some State Pension based on their earlier NI contributions. The State Pension is not awarded automatically except in the circumstances described above – you have to make a claim. So if you think you may be entitled to a State Pension, and you have not been contacted about making a claim, contact The Pension Service. However, you should be aware that if you are already receiving a State Pension or another benefit, such as a State Pension based on your husband's NI contributions record or a Widow's Pension, you may not be entitled to anything more.

Category B State Pensions for married men and civil partners

If your wife or your civil partner was born before 6 April 1950, then as a married man or civil partner you are not able to claim a Basic State Pension based on your wife or civil partner's NI contributions record. However, the rules have now changed so people reaching State Pension age now may be able to claim.

After 6 April 2010, if you reach State Pension age and you are not entitled to a Basic State Pension of at least £58.50 a week based on your own NI contributions record, you can claim a pension based on your wife or civil partner's NI contributions record if they were born on or after 6 April 1950 and have reached State Pension age. This means that husbands and female civil partners could start to qualify from May 2010 and male civil partners from April 2015. This applies regardless of when you reach State Pension age yourself.

If you qualify for a Category B State Pension as a husband or civil partner, the rules are in line with those set out above for wives.

Increases for dependants

In the past a husband has been able to claim an increase in his State Pension for a dependent wife who is under State Pension age, and in limited circumstances a wife has been able to claim for a dependent husband. The rules have now changed and from 6 April 2010 it is no longer possible to claim an increase for a dependent spouse. This also applies if you reached State Pension age before 6 April 2010 but put off claiming your State Pension until that date or later.

If you were already receiving an increase in your State Pension for a dependant at the time the new rules came into effect on 6 April 2010, you can continue to get the increase as long as you continue to meet the conditions explained below until the dependant reaches State Pension age or 5 April 2020, whichever is sooner.

Dependent wives If you are a married man aged 65 or over and were receiving the increase for your wife since before 6 April 2010 and you live together, your State Pension will be increased by a maximum of £57.05 a week. However, you will not get any increase for your wife if she gets State Pension or certain benefits of £57.05 or more a week. The increase may also be affected by any earnings she has. You will not be able to get the increase if she is

7

working and earns more than £65.45 a week (after certain expenses connected with work have been deducted). Any occupational or personal pension she gets will be counted as earnings.

If you do not live with your wife, you may be able to get the increase as set out above if you are making a contribution to her maintenance. In this situation the increase will not be paid if she earns more than £57.05 a week.

Dependent husbands If you are a married woman and have been getting the increase to your State Pension since before 6 April 2010, you will only have been able to claim the increase of up to £57.05 if you were receiving Incapacity Benefit with an additional sum for your husband immediately before you started to get the State Pension. The increase will stop if your husband has a State Pension or certain other benefits of £57.05 a week, or if he earns more than £65.45 a week (£57.05 if you do not live together).

Divorce, dissolved civil partnerships and separation

Divorced people If you are divorced but do not qualify for a full State Pension based on your own NI contributions record, you may be able to use your former spouse's contribution record to increase the amount of Basic State Pension you get to the maximum pension for a single person of £97.65 a week. You are not entitled to your former spouse's Graduated Retirement Benefit or Additional State Pension. (However, since December 2000 when rules on 'pension sharing' came into effect, it has been possible for Additional State Pension to be divided as part of a divorce settlement.)

Your former spouse's NI contributions record is substituted for your own from the start of your working life up to your divorce or just for the period of your marriage.

If you get divorced before State Pension age, you may need to pay further NI contributions after your divorce to qualify for a Basic State Pension. If you are receiving a Category B State Pension based on your husband or wife's NI contributions record, you may be able to use the rules outlined above to get a full State Pension. If you remarry or form a civil partnership before State Pension age, you cannot claim a State Pension on your former husband or wife's NI contributions record. However, if you remarry or form a civil partnership after State Pension age, you will not lose any State Pension based on your previous spouse's NI contributions record.

Dissolved civil partnerships The term 'dissolution' is used if civil partners legally separate; it is the equivalent of divorce for married couples. State Pension rules are the same as those described here for divorced people.

Separation If you are separated from your husband, wife or civil partner and you do not qualify for a Basic State Pension on your own NI contributions record when you reach State Pension age, or you are entitled only to a State Pension of less than £58.50 a week, you may be able to claim a Category B Basic State Pension of up to £58.50 a week when your spouse or civil partner reaches State Pension age – see pages 6–7. As explained there, before 5 April 2010 this only applied to married women and for husbands and civil partners it depended on the date of birth of their wife or partner.

State Pensions for widows and widowers and surviving civil partners

This section looks at the amount of State Pension that a widow, widower or surviving civil partner can get at State Pension age. For information about bereavement benefits for people under State Pension age, see pages 156–158. Some aspects of the rules are different for widowers and civil partners who reached State Pension age before April

2010. These are covered briefly below. Contact The Pension Service or a local advice agency if you need further information.

Widows If you were under State Pension age when your husband died and you have not remarried or formed a civil partnership, you may be entitled to the State Pension based on your late husband's NI contributions record and/or your own, once you reach State Pension age. The amount you get will depend upon your own, and your late husband's, NI contributions record and the age at which you were widowed. If you had reached State Pension age when your husband died, and were not getting the full Basic State Pension, you may be able to use his NI contributions record to bring your Basic State Pension up to a maximum of £97.65 a week.

You may also get Additional State Pension and/or Graduated Retirement Benefit based on your husband's NI contributions record, as explained on pages 26–27 and 28.

Once you are getting the State Pension at age 60 or over, you can remarry, form a civil partnership or live with a partner without losing a State Pension based on your previous husband's NI contributions record.

Widowers and surviving civil partners If you reach State Pension age on or after 6 April 2010, the inheritance rules are the same as those described above for widows. If you reached State Pension age before 6 April 2010 and were bereaved on or after 6 April 1979 and do not have enough NI contributions of your own, you may be entitled to a State Pension based on your wife or civil partner's NI contributions record, provided you were both over State Pension age when they died. You may also inherit some of your wife/civil partner's Additional State Pension and/or Graduated Retirement Benefit, as explained on pages 26–27 and 28. If you were bereaved under State Pension age on or after 9 April 2001, the rules are the same as for widows.

If you do not fulfil the above conditions, perhaps because your late wife or civil partner died before State Pension age when you had already reached that age before 6 April 2010, you may in some circumstances be able to use your wife/civil partner's NI contributions record in order to increase your Basic State Pension up to a maximum of £97.65 a week.

You may also get Additional State Pension based on your wife/civil partner's contribution record (see pages 26–27).

Once you are receiving a State Pension you will not lose any State Pension based on your former wife/civil partner's contributions if you remarry or enter a civil partnership.

The contribution conditions

This section explains the contribution conditions for the Basic State Pension. Your contribution record will depend on the NI contributions you have paid, any 'credits' you received and any HRP you received for tax years before 2010/11. Changes to the contribution conditions were introduced on 6 April 2010. In this section we explain the rules for people who reached State Pension age on or before 5 April 2010 and also the new rules that will apply to people who reach State Pension age on or after 6 April 2010.

Both men and women aged 80 or over who have not paid enough contributions for a Basic State Pension might qualify for the non-contributory State Pension described on page 34.

If you reached State Pension age on or before 5 April 2010

If you reached State Pension age on or before 5 April 2010, there are two conditions that you must meet to get a State Pension. The first condition is that you have paid sufficient contributions during at least one year in your working life since 6 April 1975 or paid at least 50 flat-rate NI contributions at any time before 6 April 1975. Credited contributions cannot count towards this first condition.

The second condition is that to get a full Basic State Pension you must normally have paid or been credited with NI contributions for 90% of the years of your 'working life'. Your working life normally starts in the tax year (i.e. 6 April to 5 April) when you were 16 and ends with the last full tax year before you reached State Pension age (60 for women born on or before 5 April 1950, 65 for men). Each year in your working life that you have paid or been credited with sufficient NI contributions is called a 'qualifying year'. (See below for more information about what is meant by a qualifying year.)

A woman who reached State Pension age before 6 April 2010, and had a working life of 44 years, will get a full Basic State Pension if 39 of the years are qualifying years. A man who reached State Pension age before 6 April 2010 and had a working life of 49 years will get a full Basic State Pension if he has 44 qualifying years.

If you are not entitled to the full Basic State Pension, you may get a reduced one. So, for example, if you have half the number of years needed, your pension will be half the normal rate. However, to get any Basic State Pension at all you must have a minimum number of years' NI contributions (normally 10 for a woman or 11 for a man).

If you reach State Pension age on or after 6 April 2010

Both men and women who reach State Pension age on or after 6 April 2010 will receive the full Basic State Pension if they have 30 or more qualifying years. If you have fewer than 30 qualifying years, you will get a reduced Basic State Pension as long as you have at least one qualifying year. You do not need to have a minimum number of qualifying years and there is no longer a requirement that at least one of your qualifying years needs to be based on paid NI contributions (as opposed to credited NI contributions).

Getting a forecast

If you are more than 30 days away from State Pension age, you can get a forecast to check whether you have paid enough contributions to get a full State Pension.

TO APPLY FOR A STATE PENSION FORECAST, complete form BR19, which is obtainable from the State Pension Forecasting Team on 0845 300 0168 or using the online service on the Direct Gov website (www.direct.gov.uk).

Paid NI contributions

If you have earnings of £97 a week or more (the level of the 'Lower Earnings Limit' in 2010/11), you will be building up entitlement to the Basic State Pension. However, you do not start to pay NI contributions until your earnings reach £110 a week. If you have earnings of between £97 and £110, you will be treated as though you are paying NI contributions and will still be building up entitlement to the Basic State Pension and other contributory benefits. When reference is made in this book to people who have 'paid' NI contributions, this includes people with earnings between £97 and £110 a week who will not actually be paying NI but are still treated as having paid NI contributions.

How are contributions paid?   Since April 1975 employed people have paid contributions as a percentage of earnings, and these are collected with Income Tax. Self-employed people pay flat-rate contributions each week and these count towards the Basic State Pension. If your taxable income is over a certain amount, extra contributions will be collected with your Income Tax.

Reduced-rate married woman's contributions At one time as a married woman or widow you were able to choose to pay reduced-rate contributions. These do not count towards a State Pension in your own right and it is not possible to pay voluntary contributions or get HRP to make up any gaps in your contribution record for years when you were paying or had the right to pay reduced-rate contributions. Married women in this position will usually not be eligible for credits either.

Working abroad Contributions made abroad may help you qualify for the Basic State Pension if you worked in another European Union country or one that has a reciprocal agreement with the UK.

Qualifying years A 'qualifying year' is a tax year in which you have paid or been credited with enough NI contributions to go towards a State Pension. Since 1978 a 'qualifying year' has been one in which NI contributions are paid on earnings that are the same as, or more than, 52 times the weekly Lower Earnings Limit. (Between April 1975 and April 1978 the qualifying earnings were 50 times the Lower Earnings Limit.) This tax year, 2010/11, the Lower Earnings Limit is £97 a week.

Before 1975 working people paid NI contributions by weekly stamp. To work out your qualifying years before 1975, all your stamps (paid and credited) are added up and divided by 50, rounding up any that are left over – but you cannot have more qualifying years worked out in this way than the number of years in your working life up to April 1975.

Credits If you are under State Pension age you may get a credit in place of an NI contribution in certain circumstances. For example, you will get a credit for each week you register for Jobseeker's Allowance and are seeking work or you are unable to work because you are sick or disabled or you are receiving Carer's Allowance.

Men aged 60–64 who were born on or before 5 October 1950 who are not paying contributions will normally get credits automatically even if they are not ill or signing on as unemployed. These credits will be gradually phased out for men who reach age 60 after 5 October 2010. So, for example, if you were born between 6 October 1950 and 5 October 1951, you can get a maximum of four years of automatic credits. You cannot get these automatic credits for any tax year during which you are abroad for more than six months.

Credits for parents and carers from 6 April 2010

From 6 April 2010 HRP (see below) has been replaced by weekly credits for parents and carers. You get a credit for each week that you fulfil certain caring conditions, including receiving Child Benefit for a child under the age of 12 or being an approved foster carer. There is also a new Carer's Credit available for those providing care for at least 20 hours a week for one or more sick or disabled persons who get Attendance Allowance (AA) or Constant Attendance Allowance or the middle or highest rate of the care component of Disability Living Allowance (DLA), or whose need for care has been certified by a health or social care professional. You will need to make an application to get credits in this situation. You will also need to apply for the credits given to foster parents, in which case you should do so before the end of the tax year following the one in which you consider you are entitled to credits. Late applications can sometimes be accepted if there is a good reason for not applying earlier. However, you do not need to apply for credits awarded because you are receiving Child Benefit or Carer's Allowance.

Credits for parents and carers can be combined with paid contributions and other credits to make a full qualifying year whereas under the previous system of HRP you could get HRP only if you met the conditions throughout a full tax year. If you reach State Pension age on or after 6 April 2010, any full years of HRP you have been awarded will be converted to a year of credits up to a maximum of 22 years.

In the 2009 Budget the Chancellor announced that, in the future, grandparents or other adult family members caring for 20 hours or more for a child in the family aged 12 or under will be able to get credits towards their Basic State Pension. This is due to come into effect from April 2011.

Late and voluntary NI contributions   If there are periods when you will not be paying NI contributions, perhaps because you will be abroad, you may want to consider paying NI voluntary contributions to protect your NI contributions record. If there are gaps in your NI contribution record, it is sometimes possible to pay late contributions. But note that for people reaching State Pension age on or after 6 April 2010 the rules have changed so that you need only 30 years of NI contributions to get a full Basic State Pension (see pages 12–13).

Voluntary NI contributions must normally be paid by the end of the sixth tax year after the one in which they are due. After the tax year has ended, people are usually contacted if they have gaps in their NI contribution record and invited to pay voluntary NI contributions.

However, in 2008 the Government announced new provisions to allow some people to pay up to six years of voluntary NI contributions on top of the normal provisions to fill gaps going back to 1975/76. This applies to people who reach State Pension age between 6 April 2008 and 5 April 2015 who already have at least 20 qualifying years.

It is often a good idea to get advice if you are not sure whether you will benefit from paying voluntary contributions, as it can be quite complicated. Contact HM Revenue & Customs (HMRC, previously the Inland Revenue) or a local advice agency.

Home Responsibilities Protection

HRP started in 1978 to protect the NI contribution record of people caring for a child or a sick or disabled person. It helps protect your Basic State Pension and bereavement benefits for your spouse or civil partner, and since 6 April 2002 may help you build up Additional State Pension through the State Second Pension (see pages 23–24). In April 2010 it was replaced by the new credits for parents and carers, as explained above. If you reach State Pension age on 6 April 2010 or later, any years of HRP you have been awarded will be converted into a year of credits (up to a maximum of 22 years).

You cannot get HRP for the years when you were looking after someone before April 1978.

You may get HRP if you worked and paid full NI contributions for part of the year before 2010/11 but not enough to count as a qualifying year. However, a married woman or widow cannot get HRP for any tax year in which she would only be due to pay reduced-rate NI contributions, if she was working.

You are entitled to HRP if you meet any of the following conditions, or in some situations a combination of them, for a whole tax year before 2010/11 (but note that the rules changed for the third condition):

- You received Child Benefit for a child under 16.
- You received Income Support and you were substantially engaged in looking after a sick or disabled person.
- For at least 35 hours a week you looked after someone who received, for a minimum of 48 weeks in the year, AA, the middle or highest rate of the care component of DLA, or Constant Attendance Allowance. For tax years before 6 April 1994, the allowance had to be paid for 52 weeks.

- You were a registered foster parent (for years from 2003/04 onwards).

If you get Carer's Allowance, you will normally be getting NI credits towards your State Pension, so you will not need HRP, although you cannot get credits or HRP if you retained the right to pay the married woman's reduced-rate contributions.

How to work it out

For people reaching State Pension age before 6 April 2010 HRP makes it easier for you to qualify for a Basic State Pension. Each year of 'home responsibility' will be taken away from the number of qualifying years you need to get a full Basic State Pension. However, HRP cannot be used to reduce the number of qualifying years to below 20.

For example: if you are a woman who reached the age of 60 before 6 April 2010 and you had 10 years of HRP, you will get a full Basic State Pension if you have 29 years of NI contributions rather than the normal 39 years.

When to apply

HRP should be given automatically if you qualify under the first two conditions described above. You should not have to apply for it.

You must apply for HRP if you qualify under the third or fourth condition – because you were looking after someone who was getting one of the allowances mentioned above, such as AA, or because you were a foster parent – or if you qualified under one condition for part of the tax year and under another for the rest of the year.

Applications for HRP in respect of years spent caring for a sick or disabled person before 2002/03 can be made at any time up to State Pension age. However, for years from April

2002 onwards, you will need to apply by the end of the third year following the year for which you want HRP. For example, for caring during the 2007/08 tax year you should apply between 6 April 2008 and 5 April 2011. Ask for leaflet CF411 from HM Revenue & Customs; it is also available online (www.hmrc.gov.uk/forms/cf411.pdf).

How to claim your State Pension

About four months before you reach State Pension age you should be sent a claim pack. You can ring 0800 731 7898 to make a claim over the phone or to ask for a claim form. You can also claim online. If you have not been contacted about claiming your State Pension three months before your birthday, contact The Pension Service or ring 0800 731 7898. If you are making a claim on your spouse or civil partner's contributions, you will need to make a separate claim.

You may decide to put off claiming your State Pension at that time in order to get extra State Pension or a lump-sum payment. This is also known as 'deferring' your State Pension and is explained on pages 28–34. If you do put off claiming the State Pension, contact The Pension Service well in advance of when you want to start claiming it.

How your State Pension is paid

Most people now get their State Pension by direct payment into an account. When you apply for your State Pension you will be given information about the different types of bank, building society and Post Office accounts you can use. People who reached State Pension age before 6 April 2010 had the option to get their State Pension paid weekly in advance or four-weekly or quarterly. The position has changed for people who reach State Pension age from 6 April 2010 onwards, when weekly payments will be in arrears and people who previously received a working age benefit paid two-weekly in arrears will normally continue to be paid in this way.

If you cannot manage an account or you do not provide account details, you will be sent a weekly cheque in the post. You can sign the back of the cheque to authorise someone else to collect your State Pension at the Post Office. If, for example, you have different carers collecting your State Pension, this may be the best way of getting your money each week. Although cheques will be phased out in the future, the Government has said that this will not happen until there is a suitable replacement system that will meet the needs of those who cannot use an account. There are also ways of authorising someone else to collect your money from a Post Office, or a bank or building society account.

When you are deciding how to have your State Pension paid, consider the different options – if you are unsure, a local advice agency may be able to help.

> FOR MORE INFORMATION, see Age UK factsheet The State Pension, which is available from Age UK Advice on 0800 169 65 65.

Pay-day for anyone who started to get their State Pension before 28 September 1984 is normally Thursday. For people who retired after that date and before April 2010, pay-day is usually Monday, although if your spouse is already receiving a State Pension on Thursday, you can choose to have yours on the same day. From April 2010 the State Pension pay-day will be based on your NI number and could be any weekday. Payments used to be made only for full weeks and your State Pension would start from your first pay-day after you were entitled to payment. However from 6 April 2010 it is possible to get a part-week payment if you were previously receiving a working age benefit which stops before your State Pension starts to be paid. Most State Pensions of £5 a week or less are paid once a year, in December, in arrears. If you ask for payment by Direct Payment, you will be paid by that method; otherwise you will be sent a cheque.

Going abroad or living there If you get your payment by weekly cheque, you must cash this within one month of the date shown on it. If you are going abroad for longer than this (or for a shorter period but do not want the cheques sent while you are away), contact The Pension Service well in advance to discuss how to receive your money when you return. If your pension is paid into an account, you do not need to tell The Pension Service unless you are staying abroad for more than six months.

If you are going abroad for some time, you can arrange to get your State Pension in the country where you are staying. If you remain abroad, the annual State Pension increase will be paid only if you are living in a European Union country or in a country with which the UK has special arrangements.

FOR MORE INFORMATION, contact your pension centre or the International Pension Centre, The Pension Service, Tyneview Park, Whitley Road, Benton, Newcastle upon Tyne NE98 1BA. Tel: 0191 218 7777.

Going into hospital Before April 2005 your State Pension could be reduced after a period of time in hospital. But the rules were changed, and now your State Pension will continue to be paid however long you are in hospital. If you are receiving benefits such as AA, these may still be affected by a hospital stay.

FOR MORE INFORMATION, see Department for Work and Pensions (DWP) leaflet DWP1029 Going into Hospital?, which is available from the DWP website (www.dwp.gov.uk).

If you disagree with a decision

If you think that you have been awarded the wrong amount of State Pension, or disagree with another decision to do with your State Pension, you can either ask for the decision to be revised or appeal against it. Further details are given on pages 41–44.

ADDITIONAL STATE PENSION

This scheme started on 6 April 1978. From 1978 to April 2002, Additional State Pension was built up under the State Earnings-Related Pension Scheme (SERPS, see below) but since April 2002 the Additional State Pension has been built up under the State Second Pension (S2P).

When you get your State Pension you may get Additional State Pension on top of your Basic State Pension, or you may qualify for an Additional State Pension even if you do not get any Basic State Pension. The Additional State Pension is taxable.

The Additional State Pension is based on earnings, and on any credited earnings that some carers and long-term sick or disabled people have been entitled to following the introduction of the S2P in April 2002. However, you do not build up any Additional State Pension based on your earnings if you are self-employed, paying the reduced-rate married woman's contributions, or earning less than the Lower Earnings Limit (which is £97 a week in 2010/11). Employees may also be contracted out of the State scheme, as explained below.

The Additional State Pension is related to your weekly earnings between the weekly Lower and Upper Accrual Point (£97 and £770 respectively in 2010/11), or credited earnings under the S2P, from April 1978 until the 5th of the April before you reach State Pension age (see page 3). These earnings are revalued in line with increases in average earnings.

SERPS

If you reached State Pension age before 6 April 1999, your total revalued earnings were divided by 80 to give the yearly amount of Additional State Pension. This formula provides an Additional State Pension based on 25% of earnings between the specified levels.

However, changes were introduced to phase in, between 1999 and 2009, reductions to the amount of Additional State Pension people get. The main aim of these changes was to reduce the maximum level of SERPS from 25% of earnings to 20% for people reaching State Pension age from 2009 onwards (with some protection for years up to 1987/88). However, as explained below, the S2P provides a more generous pension to people with low or modest earnings.

State Second Pension

Since 6 April 2002 the Additional State Pension has been built up under the S2P. If you have entitlement under SERPS, this will be protected, so if you reached State Pension age on or after 6 April 2003, you may get an Additional State Pension built up partly under SERPS and partly under the S2P.

Like SERPS, the S2P can provide an Additional State Pension based on your earnings (although in the future it will start to move to becoming a flat-rate pension). However, it is calculated in a way that is more beneficial to those with low or modest earnings.

For this tax year, 2010/11, employees with annual earnings of at least £5,044 but less than £14,100 will be treated as though they have earnings of £14,100.

For years 2002/03 to 2009/10 you will be treated as though you have earnings of £14,100 if, throughout the year, you were entitled to:

- Carer's Allowance.
- The long-term rate of Incapacity Benefit (or would have been if you had satisfied the contribution conditions) or Severe Disablement Allowance or, in some circumstances, Employment and Support Allowance. (For people who reached State Pension age before 6 April 2010 credits for those receiving disability benefits were subject to having made a

certain number of years of contributions on retirement).

- HRP (see pages 17–19) because you were looking after a long-term sick or disabled person or a child under the age of six.

Usually people will be credited into the S2P automatically, although some people need to claim HRP – when this is the case since 2002/03 you have needed to do this by the end of the third year following the year for which you are claiming HRP.

To qualify for a year of the S2P for years before April 2010 you must fulfil one of the criteria for a whole tax year – for example, you cannot combine different types of caring responsibilities, or be providing care for part of the year and fulfil the disability conditions for the rest of the year.

For years from April 2010/11 onwards

From this tax year (2010/11) onwards, it will be easier for disabled people and those providing care to build up the S2P. A qualifying year for S2P can now be built up using the new Carer Credit, credits linked to disability benefits, NI contributions from earnings or through a combination of credits and contributions based on earnings. The conditions for the Carer Credit are the same as for the credit for the Basic State Pension (see pages 15–16).

Contracting out of the State Second Pension

'Contracting out' means that you give up your entitlement to Additional State Pension by joining an occupational pension scheme, a stakeholder pension scheme or another type of personal pension scheme. These schemes have to satisfy certain conditions in order for you to contract out of the State scheme.

If you contract out through your employer's occupational pension scheme, this will provide a pension in place of the

Additional State Pension, and both you and your employer will pay a lower rate of NI contributions. If your employer's occupational scheme is not contracted out, both you and your employer will pay full-rate NI contributions and you will build up entitlement to both the full Additional State Pension and the pension due under the rules of your employer's scheme. An adjustment may be made to your occupational pension in respect of any Additional State Pension that you build up during the period that you are a member of your employer's scheme. Contact your employer or the scheme administrator if you need more information.

If you contract out with a personal pension or a stakeholder pension, once a year HM Revenue & Customs will pay a rebate of your NI contributions direct to your pension provider, together with tax relief at the basic rate on your share of the rebate. These payments are known as 'Minimum Contributions'.

> FOR MORE INFORMATION, see HM Revenue & Customs leaflet CA17 Employee's Guide to Minimum Contributions. Copies are available only on the HM Revenue & Customs website (www.hmrc.gov.uk).

Anyone with a personal or stakeholder pension earning below £14,100 in the 2010/11 tax year will get a 'top-up' of the Additional State Pension irrespective of whether or not they are contracted out. Anyone in an occupational pension scheme earning between £5,044 and around £32,200 will get a 'top-up' of the Additional State Pension.

It is a good idea to seek professional financial advice before contracting out, especially if you are considering entering a money-purchase scheme or taking out an appropriate personal pension. It is also important that you continue to review your pension arrangements on a regular basis to ensure that you are making adequate provision for your retirement. Again, you should take advice. Remember, though, that if you choose to see an adviser, you may have to pay for their advice.

For the period April 1978 to April 1997 any estimate of the amount of State Pension that you will get when you retire will show how much Additional State Pension you have built up during that period. If you were contracted out of SERPS for any time, the statement will show a 'contracted-out deduction', which takes into account the period when you were not paying into SERPS. The amount of Additional State Pension (before the deduction) minus the contracted-out deduction shows how much Additional State Pension will actually be paid on top of your Basic State Pension.

If you are contracted out, you will not build up any Additional State Pension entitlement after 6 April 1997.

Widows, widowers and surviving civil partners

When a widow starts to get her State Pension or if she is already receiving her State Pension at the time she is widowed, she can inherit all or some of her late husband's Additional State Pension (adjusted for periods when he was contracted out of SERPS/S2P). As a widow any amount you are entitled to is added to any Additional State Pension on your own contributions up to the maximum amount of Additional State Pension a single person could get. Subject to this maximum level, the amount of SERPS pension you can inherit depends on when your husband dies and when he reaches, or was due to reach, State Pension age (65). A woman whose husband died on or before 5 October 2002 inherits his entire SERPS pension. She can also inherit his entire SERPS pension if he dies after that date but was born on or before 5 October 1937 (and therefore reached State Pension age on or before 5 October 2002).

If your husband's date of birth is between 6 October 1937 and 5 October 1945, you will be able to inherit between 60% and 90% of his SERPS pension, depending on his precise date of birth. If he is due to reach State Pension age on or after 6 October 2010, you will only be able to inherit 50% of his SERPS pension.

For widowers or civil partners who reach State Pension age on or after 6 April 2010 the rules are similar to those set out above for widows. In this case the widower or civil partner can inherit some or all of their wife/partner's SERPS, depending on when they reach State Pension age. They will be able to inherit all their wife/partner's SERPS pension (subject to the maximum level) if the wife/partner died on or before 5 October 2002, or if they die after that date but had already reached State Pension age by 5 October 2002.

Widowers or civil partners who reached State Pension age before 6 April 2010 may also be able to inherit their spouse/partner's SERPS, but generally this is only possible if both partners had reached State Pension age at the time of bereavement. As explained earlier, for contributions made since April 2002, SERPS has been replaced by the S2P. The maximum amount of the S2P that a widow, widower or surviving civil partner can inherit is 50%, regardless of when they are widowed.

FOR MORE INFORMATION, see leaflet SERPSL1, which provides information about inheritance of SERPS and can be obtained from the Pension Information Ordering Line 0845 731 3233.

GRADUATED RETIREMENT BENEFIT

This taxable pension scheme, sometimes called 'Graduated Pension', existed from April 1961 to April 1975 and was based on graduated contributions paid from earnings. If you were over 18 during this period and paying graduated contributions, your weekly Graduated Retirement Benefit for the year 2010/11 will be 11.53p for every £9.00 of contributions paid.

The rates used to be different for men and women but from 6 April 2010 they have been equalised. This will be paid when you claim your State Pension, normally with the Basic State Pension. However, you can get Graduated Retirement Benefit even if you do not qualify for a Basic State Pension.

Married women, widows, widowers and surviving civil partners

A widow can inherit half her late husband's Graduated Retirement Benefit whether she is over or under State Pension age at the time of bereavement. The rules are now the same for a widower or surviving civil partner who reaches State Pension age on or after 6 April 2010.

A widower or surviving civil partner who reached State Pension age before 5 April 2010 and whose wife/civil partner died after 5 April 1979 can inherit half their late spouse or civil partner's Graduated Retirement Benefit, provided they were both over State Pension age when the late wife/civil partner died.

PUTTING OFF CLAIMING YOUR STATE PENSION

Once you reach State Pension age you can get your State Pension if you satisfy the contribution conditions even if you are still working. Alternatively, you can choose to put off claiming your State Pension, in which case you can get extra State Pension or a one-off taxable lump-sum payment at a later date. Putting off claiming your State Pension is also described as 'deferral'.

If you put off claiming your State Pension for at least seven weeks before 6 April 2005, it is increased for that period by about 7.5% for each year you put off claiming. However, under current rules, which were introduced on 6 April 2005, your State Pension will be increased by about 10.4% for each full year you do not claim it or, instead of receiving extra State Pension, you can choose to receive a lump-sum payment along with your normal State Pension. Both the current rules and the old rules are summarised here. If you put off claiming both before and after April 2005, your State Pension will be increased according to the old rules until April 2005 and then, for the period you put off claiming after April 2005, according to the new rules.

Before April 2005 people could put off claiming their State Pension for a maximum of five years – so they could normally put off claiming their State Pension only up to the age of 65 for women or 70 for men (although there were circumstances when a married woman of 65 or over could put off claiming her State Pension if she had a husband under 70 who put off claiming his State Pension). Under the rules from April 2005 onwards, there are no time limits for how long you can put off claiming, so, if you wish, you can put off claiming your State Pension for more than five years.

You do not have to be working to put off claiming your State Pension but you cannot be counted as putting off claiming your State Pension if you are receiving certain other benefits instead. For example, someone who is in receipt of Carer's Allowance and has not claimed their State Pension will not gain any extra State Pension. In addition, if you are receiving an income-related benefit, such as Pension Credit, any State Pension you put off claiming may be taken into account as notional income when calculating your entitlement. You should also note that if you are entitled to an increase for a dependant (for example, because you are a married man with a wife aged under 60) and you put off claiming your State Pension, you will not get any extra State Pension or lump sum for this part of your State Pension.

If you do claim your State Pension, it is possible to change your mind and put off claiming it instead. However, this can be done only once, and you must be living in the UK (there are exemptions to this rule for people living in the European Union and other European Economic Area (EEA) countries). So, for example, if you are claiming your State Pension (and have not claimed and then given it up before), you could choose to stop receiving it and put off claiming it for a time in order to benefit from the rules. Before April 2010 if you were married or in a civil partnership and your spouse or partner was getting a State Pension based on your contributions, you needed their consent before cancelling your State Pension, as your spouse or partner had to give up their pension too. From April 2010 this will no longer apply – they can get their Category B pension independently.

Increased Basic State Pension for periods before April 2005

If you put off claiming your State Pension for at least seven weeks before April 2005, when you do choose to claim it, your State Pension will be increased by about 7.5% a year for each full year that you did not claim it. (If you put off claiming your State Pension before 6 April 1979, you will have earned a smaller increase.) For each week that you put off claiming your State Pension, it will be increased by one-seventh of 1% – this works out as 1% for each seven weeks.

Someone who put off claiming their State Pension for the full five years will have had it increased by about 37.5%.

Putting off claiming your State Pension after April 2005

Under the current rules, if you put off claiming your State Pension for at least five weeks it will be increased by one-fifth of 1% for each week you put off claiming – this works out as 1% for each five weeks. Your State Pension will be increased by around 10.4% for each full year that you do not claim it – so, if you put off claiming your State Pension for five years, it will be increased by just over half. Alternatively, instead of extra State Pension you could get a taxable lump-sum payment plus your weekly State Pension paid at the normal rate. The lump sum will be calculated based on the amount of State Pension (excluding any State Pension increase for an adult dependant) you have forgone and a compounded interest rate of 2% above the Bank of England base rate. You have to put off claiming your State Pension for at least 12 consecutive months to have the choice of a lump-sum payment. As explained above, you will not build up entitlement to extra State Pension or a lump-sum payment if you get certain other benefits or another category of State Pension while you put off claiming your State Pension.

Even if you do not put off claiming your State Pension for a full year, you can get extra State Pension (as long as you put off claiming it for at least five weeks), or you can get your State Pension backdated to the time when you could have started to get it (but without any interest payments).

Increased Additional State Pension and Graduated Retirement Benefit

If you put off claiming your State Pension, your Additional State Pension and Graduated Retirement Benefit will be increased in the same way as the Basic State Pension; or if you opt for a lump-sum payment, they will be included in the calculation of this.

FOR MORE INFORMATION, see Pension Service leaflet NP46 and SPD2 Deferring your State Pension, *or the longer guide SPD1* Your Guide to State Pension Deferral.

People receiving a State Pension on their spouse/partner's contribution

If you are a married woman entitled to a State Pension (or an increase to your State Pension) based on your husband's contributions, from 6 April 2010, you can choose to claim this even if he is putting off claiming his State Pension. Before then you had to wait until he claimed his State Pension. Alternatively, you can also put off claiming your State Pension and when you do claim it you will get extra State Pension (or a lump sum).

In general, you will not get extra State Pension or a lump-sum payment for putting off claiming the State Pension from your husband's contributions if, while your husband is putting off claiming his State Pension, you claim any State Pension you are entitled to on your own contributions, or certain other benefits. It may be better not to claim your own State Pension (for example, if this is a small amount) if your husband is putting off claiming his State Pension. However, following a change in the rules on 6 April 2006, if you claim Graduated Retirement Benefit only, it will not stop you getting extra State Pension or a lump-sum payment from your husband's contributions.

Husbands and civil partners who reach(ed) State Pension age on or after 6 April 2010 may now also be able to get a State Pension based on their wife/civil partner's contributions once the wife/civil partner reaches State Pension age (see details on pages 6–7). The rules set out above for married women also apply to husbands and civil partners in this position.

Inheritance and divorce

If you die while you are still putting off claiming your State Pension, your surviving spouse or civil partner may be entitled to extra State Pension or a lump-sum payment when they claim their own State Pension. If you are unmarried and not in a civil partnership at the time of your death, the extra State Pension or lump sum cannot be passed on to anyone else.

If you are entitled to a shared Additional State Pension (resulting from the sharing of a former spouse or civil partner's Additional State Pension following divorce or dissolution of a civil partnership), you can also put off claiming this.

FOR MORE INFORMATION, see Pension Service guide SPD1 Your Guide to State Pension Deferral or look on the Direct Gov website (www.direct.gov.uk).

Income Tax and the impact on income-related benefits

The State Pension is taxable and is taken into account for benefits such as Pension Credit, Housing Benefit and Council Tax Benefit. If you get extra State Pension following putting off claiming, this will count as part of your taxable income and may reduce the amount of any income-related benefits you get. However, the lump-sum payment will be ignored if you claim Pension Credit, Housing Benefit or Council Tax Benefit. The lump sum will be taxed at the rate you are currently paying Income Tax on other income (so it will not put you into a higher tax band). You can choose to delay receiving it until the tax year after you start receiving your State Pension, which may be an advantage if your income is lower then.

Deciding what to do

In the past most people chose to claim their State Pension at State Pension age but the more generous rules now may mean that more people will think about putting off claiming State Pension. This may not be right for everyone, and the amount you could get will depend on your circumstances. If you are interested in putting off claiming your State Pension, it is important to find out more before you decide. Make sure you have full information and get advice if you are not sure about the different options.

FOR MORE INFORMATION, see Pension Service guide SPD1 Your Guide to State Pension Deferral, *which gives information about putting off claiming your State Pension and the things to consider, and Age UK factsheet* The State Pension, *which is available from Age UK Advice on 0800 169 65 65.*

OVER-80 STATE PENSION

This is a non-contributory taxable State Pension of £58.50 a week for people aged 80 or over who have no State Pension. (It is officially called a 'Category D' State Pension.) For someone who already gets a State Pension of less than £58.50 a week, an Over-80 State Pension can also be paid to bring that State Pension up to £58.50 a week. To qualify for this State Pension you have to be living in the UK on the day you are 80 or the date of your claim if this is later, and to have been in the UK for 10 years or more in any 20-year period after your 60th birthday. If you have lived in Gibraltar or in another European Union country, this may help you satisfy the conditions.

The Over-80 State Pension will be counted as income in full for the purposes of Pension Credit, Housing Benefit and Council Tax Benefit.

FOR MORE INFORMATION, see DWP claim form (with notes) BR2488.

ENTITLEMENTS BEFORE AND AFTER STATE PENSION AGE

The earliest age at which someone can get their State Pension is not necessarily the age at which they retire from work. Some people will stop work before State Pension age and some will work longer, while others may want to retire gradually – for example, by reducing their hours rather than leaving work completely. This section summarises the financial support available for people who are not working before State Pension age or who work after that age, referring to other parts of the book where appropriate.

If you are under State Pension age

You cannot get your State Pension until you reach State Pension age. However, you may be entitled to other financial support, as summarised here.

If you are working   Working Tax Credit can provide additional financial help to people with low incomes who work at least 16 hours a week. (See pages 150–151 for more information.) You may also be entitled to help with your housing costs from Housing Benefit and/or Council Tax Benefit.

If you are looking for work   If you are able to work and actively seeking a job, you may be entitled to Jobseeker's Allowance, as explained on pages 151–154. You may also be entitled to help with your housing costs from Housing Benefit and/or Council Tax Benefit.

If you are unable to work   If you are unable to work because of sickness, you may be entitled to Employment and Support Allowance (ESA; previously Incapacity Benefit), depending on your contribution record (see pages 115–121). You may also get ESA if you are sick and have a low income. If you are a carer, you may be entitled to Carer's Allowance (see pages 110–115). Other people under State Pension age who are not required to 'sign on' for work in order to get benefit may be entitled to Income

35

Support if they have a low income. People over the age at which women can get their State Pension can get Pension Credit without having to be available for work. You may also be entitled to help with your housing costs from Housing Benefit and/or Council Tax Benefit.

Occupational and personal pensions You may qualify for some occupational pension before State Pension age if you retire early – check with your employer for details.

You can usually claim a personal pension or stakeholder pension at any time between the ages of 55 and 75. However, if you were contracted out of SERPS/S2P, you cannot start to get the part of your personal or stakeholder pension built up from the minimum NI contributions paid into your fund until you reach the age of 60.

Protecting your State Pension If you are under State Pension age and not paying NI contributions, check that you will have enough contributions to be eligible to get a full State Pension when you reach State Pension age by contacting the HM Revenue & Customs National Insurance Contributions Office (see address on page 207).

You will get credits towards your State Pension if you are getting a benefit such as Jobseeker's Allowance, Incapacity Benefit, Employment and Support Allowance or Carer's Allowance. Men aged 60–64 may also get credits automatically even if they are not ill or signing on as unemployed although these credits are being phased out – see page 121. If you are not entitled to credits and have an incomplete NI record and you are seeking work, it may be worth signing on as unemployed even if you are not entitled to benefit – because you will get credits. Otherwise you may want to consider paying voluntary contributions.

Working after State Pension age
State Pensions Once you reach State Pension age you can choose to claim your State Pension or to put off

claiming it (in other words, 'defer' it) in order to gain later, as explained on pages 28–34. If you work and get your State Pension, it will not be affected by the amount you earn or the number of hours you work. You should note, however, that if you are claiming an increase of your State Pension for a dependent husband or wife, this increase could be affected by their earnings, as explained on pages 7–8.

Although your State Pension will not be reduced because you are working, it is counted as part of your taxable income. Your tax code will be adjusted to take into account the amount of any State Pension (including Additional State Pension and Graduated Retirement Benefit) you get.

If you carry on working after State Pension age, you will not have to pay NI contributions. You should get a 'certificate of exception' from HM Revenue & Customs to give to your employer, who will still have to pay contributions for you.

Unemployment and sickness If you have put off claiming your State Pension, you cannot claim Employment and Support Allowance or Jobseeker's Allowance if you become unable to work. This is because neither of these benefits can start to be paid to someone who has reached State Pension age.

Occupational and personal pensions If you have a private pension, you may be able to get this while you are working – contact your pension scheme for more information.

CHRISTMAS BONUS

The Christmas Bonus of £10 will be paid to people who are entitled to one of the State benefits listed below and who are living in the UK or any other European Union country during the week beginning 6 December 2010. The bonus is tax-free and has no effect on other benefits.

Who qualifies?

You will get the Christmas Bonus if you are receiving any of the following:

- a State Pension;
- Over-80 or Widow's Pension;
- AA;
- DLA (any level or component);
- Carer's Allowance;
- Industrial Death Benefit;
- Incapacity Benefit payable at the long-term rate;
- contribution-based Employment and Support Allowance (the main phase support or work components);
- Severe Disablement Allowance;
- Pension Credit;
- War Widow's Pension;
- Unemployability Supplement;
- Constant Attendance Allowance paid with a War or Industrial Injuries Disablement Benefit.

The Christmas Bonus is also payable to someone aged 65 or over who gets a War Disablement Pension but who does not get a qualifying benefit.

Only one bonus can be given to each person. However, someone over State Pension age may get an additional bonus for a dependent spouse or an unmarried partner who is over State Pension age or who reached State Pension age during the qualifying week but is not entitled to the bonus in their own right.

How it is paid

There is usually no need to claim, as the bonus is paid automatically. Depending on the way your State Pension is normally paid, the bonus will be added to your State Pension and paid into your account, or sent by cheque. If you think you are entitled to the bonus but do not receive it, contact The Pension Service or the Jobcentre Plus office that pays your State Pension or benefits.

OCCUPATIONAL AND PERSONAL PENSIONS

Occupational pensions are run by employers and are also known as 'company' pensions. Personal pensions and stakeholder pensions are provided by financial institutions, such as banks, building societies and insurance companies.

Employees earning over a certain amount must either pay into the Additional State Pension or be contracted out into an occupational, personal or stakeholder pension, as explained on pages 24–26. Self-employed people do not have access either to the Additional State Pension or to an occupational pension and cannot therefore contract out. They can, however, take out a personal pension or a stakeholder pension that is not contracted out of the State scheme.

Stakeholder pensions have been available since April 2001 and are a type of personal pension that must satisfy certain government standards with the aim of providing flexibility and value for money. Starting gradually from 2012, most employees will be automatically enrolled (with the choice to opt out) into either their workplace pension or the National Employment Savings Trust (NEST), a new scheme which is being introduced at the same time.

It is not within the scope of this book to give information about the different types of pension scheme and, in any case, terms and conditions vary. Contact your scheme provider if you need more information – for example, if you need to find out more about provision for widows or other dependants.

FOR MORE INFORMATION, if you have paid into one or more pensions in the past and have lost touch with any of the schemes, contact the Pension Tracing Service, The Pension Service, Tyneview Park, Whitley Road, Benton, Newcastle upon Tyne NE98 1BA. Tel: 0845 600 2537. Website: www.direct.gov.uk/en/ pensionsandretirementplanning

Getting advice

If you have a problem with your pension that you cannot sort out with your employer or pension provider, you can seek advice from The Pensions Advisory Service (TPAS – contact details on page 209) or a Citizens Advice Bureau. TPAS is an independent voluntary organisation with a network of local advisers who can offer free help and advice. If TPAS cannot resolve your problem, it may recommend that you make a complaint to the Pensions Ombudsman.

FOR MORE INFORMATION, see the DWP leaflets on State Pensions and other pensions. These can be obtained from the Pensions Infomation Order Line on 0845 731 3233 or the website (www.dwp.gov.uk).

How State benefits are affected

All pensions (State Pensions, occupational pensions, and personal and stakeholder pensions) will be counted as income in full for the purposes of calculating State benefits such as Pension Credit, Income Support, income-based Jobseeker's Allowance (JSA), income-related Employment and Support Allowance, Housing Benefit and Council Tax Benefit. They can also reduce the amount of contribution-based JSA you get or the amount of Incapacity Benefit or contribution-based Employment and Support Allowance paid. If you get a State Pension or benefit and claim an increase for a dependent wife or husband, any occupational, personal or stakeholder pension they get will be counted as earnings and may affect your increase, as explained on pages 7–8.

DECISION-MAKING AND APPEALS

This section outlines the system of decision-making and the way that you can challenge a decision about a State Pension or benefit. There is a different review system for the discretionary Social Fund, which is explained on pages 90–91.

When you get a letter giving details of whether you have been awarded a benefit, and if so how much, you will also get information about what to do if you disagree with the decision. It is very important to be aware that there are time limits for challenging decisions – take action as soon as possible if you are unhappy with a decision.

If you want to challenge a decision, it is often useful to get advice from a local agency, such as a Citizens Advice Bureau. For example, it may be able to advise on whether you have a good case; contact the pension centre on your behalf; prepare your case; and it may perhaps be able to represent you at an appeal tribunal.

Decisions

Most social security decisions are made by the Secretary of State – in practice by a decision-maker in the DWP on behalf of the Secretary of State. Decisions on Housing Benefit and Council Tax Benefit are made by decision-makers in the local authority. In most situations decisions can be revised or superseded or you can take the matter to an appeal tribunal. You should note, however, that the information below does not apply to certain types of decision, such as how benefits are paid. These decisions are not subject to the appeals procedures, although you can still ask for the decision to be reconsidered. For some decisions about contributions you will need to contact HM Revenue & Customs if you disagree with the decision.

Revising and superseding decisions

If you are refused benefit or disagree with the amount awarded, you have one calendar month in which to ask for the decision to be revised (in other words, to be looked at again and changed). If you have not been given a written 'statement of reasons' for the decision, you can ask for one within the one-month period, in which case the time limit will be extended by 14 days. If the statement arrives outside the one-month period, the 14 days start from when you get it. The one-month time limit can also be extended to up to 13 months in certain situations if there are 'special circumstances' for asking for a late revision.

If you are asking for the decision to be revised, send in any additional information that might help. Asking for a revision is intended to be a quick and flexible procedure. You can do this by letter or phone, explaining why you think the decision is wrong – make it clear that you are asking for your benefit to be revised. You will then be sent a letter explaining whether the decision is being revised. If you are still not happy with the decision, you can appeal (see below).

Decisions awarding benefit may also be 'superseded' at any time if, for example, your circumstances change or there is new information that affects the decision. Let the DWP know as soon as possible about any information that might affect your benefit. Otherwise you may lose benefit or get too much and have to repay money.

Appeals

If you have received a decision you disagree with, or you have asked for a decision to be revised and you are not happy with the outcome of that application, you can appeal. You should appeal within one month of the date of the decision or the letter about the revision. This time limit can be extended to up to 13 months, but you must explain why it is late. If you appeal, the decision will be looked at again to see if it can be revised. If the decision is revised in your favour, the appeal will not go ahead, even if you do not get all you asked for. You can appeal against the new decision if you are still unhappy.

Ask for an appeal, using the form attached to DWP leaflet GL24 *If you think our decision is wrong,* if possible (although other requests in writing will be accepted), saying which decision you are appealing against and giving the reasons why you disagree with the decision. You should send your appeal to the DWP office that sent you the decision notice.

When your appeal is accepted you will be sent information and papers relevant to your case. The Tribunals Service will send a form asking if you wish to attend the tribunal hearing or if you are happy for the appeal to be decided just on the basis of the written information provided. It is important that you return this form within the specified time limit or your appeal may go ahead without you. It is always better to attend if possible so that you have an opportunity to explain the position and answer questions.

Although most appeals will be considered by a tribunal, there is the option for the tribunal to 'strike out' an appeal – for example if you do not provide information requested within the specified time limits. Contact a local agency for help if this happens.

> FOR MORE INFORMATION, see DWP guide NI260 A Guide to Revision, Supersession and Appeal, which is available only on the website (www.dwp.gov.uk), or the Welfare Benefits and Tax Credits Handbook (see page 211) for more detailed information.

Tribunals

Appeals are administered by the Tribunals Service, which is an agency of the Ministry of Justice. First-tier tribunals consist of one, two or three people, depending on the benefit involved and the issues raised. Tribunal members are independent and one will be a lawyer. There may be an officer from the DWP present at the hearing.

When you arrive at the tribunal, a clerk will explain the procedures, which are intended to be as informal as possible. You will be given time to put your case and the tribunal will ask questions. The clerk should reimburse your travel expenses before you leave. The tribunal must decide whether the decision was right according to the law, but cannot change a decision just because it seems unfair. You may be told the outcome straight away; otherwise notification of the decision will be sent to you later.

If you are unhappy with the tribunal's decision, you may be able to make a further appeal to the Upper Tribunal – a local advice agency will be able to advise you how to do this.

Income-Related (Means-Tested) Benefits

This part of *Your Rights* describes the money benefits that older people may be able to claim based on their income and savings. It covers Pension Credit, Housing Benefit and Council Tax Benefit, which are weekly entitlements, and the discretionary Social Fund, which provides lump-sum payments for exceptional expenses.

Before 2010 people could claim Pension Credit when they were 60. From 6 April 2010 the age at which you can claim Pension Credit will rise in line with the increase in women's State Pension age (see chapter 1 for more details).

Qualifying age for Pension Credit to rise

As a result of the changes to the State Pension the Government is also raising the age at which a person can claim Pension Credit. From 6 April 2010 both men and women will only be able to claim Pension Credit once they have reached the age at which a woman can claim the State Pension. In this chapter we call this age 'the qualifying age for Pension Credit'.

If you were born after 6 April 1950 this age will be calculated based on your date of birth and is the same for both men and women. If you were born on or after 6 April 1955 you will not be able to claim Pension Credit until you are 65.

See chapter 1 for more details of how this date is calculated. To find out your exact Pension Credit qualifying age, call The Pension Service on 0845 606 0265 or visit the Direct Gov website (www.direct.gov.uk).

Other benefits and entitlements that were previously available to women and men at 60 (such as the higher capital disregards and the higher rates of Housing Benefit and Council Tax Benefit) will change so that they are available to both men and women at their Pension Credit qualifying age.

Pension Credit was introduced in October 2003. Although it has been widely advertised, and the Government has been encouraging older people to claim, many are still missing out. There are also around 2 million pensioners who are not claiming the Council Tax Benefit that is due to them. Homeowners are particularly likely to be missing out, perhaps because they incorrectly believe that they are not entitled to help because they own their own homes. So if you are old enough to claim, make sure that you are not missing out on the income that is due to you.

PENSION CREDIT

Pension Credit is an income-related benefit for people who have reached the qualifying age (see page 46) and who have low or modest incomes. You do not need to have paid National Insurance (NI) contributions to qualify for Pension Credit, but your income and any savings and capital over a certain level will be taken into account. Pension Credit does not have an upper capital limit. It is not taxable.

It has two parts – the Guarantee Credit and the Savings Credit. The Guarantee Credit helps with weekly basic living expenses by topping up your income to a level set by the Government. The Savings Credit provides additional cash to people aged 65 and over, who have income over a certain level from sources such as pensions and savings. People may be entitled to the Guarantee Credit or the Savings Credit, or both.

If you receive Pension Credit and you are liable to pay rent and/or Council Tax, you are also likely to qualify for Housing Benefit and/or Council Tax Benefit to help with these bills. Even if your income is too high for you to receive Pension Credit, you may still be entitled to some Housing Benefit and Council Tax Benefit. (See pages 79–90 for more information.)

Pension Credit can be paid to homeowners, tenants, and people in other circumstances such as those living with family or friends. You can work and receive Pension Credit, although most of your earnings will be taken into account. Once you get Pension Credit, you may also be able to apply for other benefits such as lump-sum payments from the Social Fund (see page 90), while if you are entitled to the Guarantee Credit this will 'passport' you to help with health costs such as a contribution towards glasses (see page 181) and free dental treatment (see pages 180–181).

People under State Pension age who are seeking work may be entitled to Jobseeker's Allowance (JSA) (see pages 151–154), while those under the qualifying age who are not able to work, for example due to caring responsibilities or incapacity, may be entitled to Income Support (see pages 154–156) or income-related Employment and Support Allowance (ESA) (see page 119). This book does not provide detailed information about the income-related benefits available to people under the qualifying age for Pension Credit, so if you need further information, contact a local advice agency or Jobcentre Plus office.

Who qualifies?

You may receive Pension Credit if you fulfil all the following conditions:

- You have reached the qualifying age for Pension Credit. As explained above this is linked to the earliest age at which women can get their State Pension, which is gradually increasing from 60 to 65 by April 2020 (you have to be 65 or over to receive Savings Credit).
- Your income is below a certain level.
- You are present and habitually resident in the UK and you are not excluded from claiming benefit because of your immigration status. Contact a local advice agency if you need further advice about the benefit position for people who have been living abroad.

Couples   For a couple, one of you applies on behalf of both partners – the person who applies must have reached Pension Credit qualifying age, although their partner can be younger. For Savings Credit at least one of a couple must have reached 65. A 'partner' is the person you are married to or living with as if you are married, or your civil partner, or the person you are living with as if you are civil partners. If you live with someone who is not your partner – such as a friend or a brother or sister – you are assessed separately.

How to work it out

To work out whether you are entitled to Pension Credit, take the following steps, which are explained in detail below:

1 Add up the value of your savings and, if you have more than £10,000, work out the 'assumed income'.

2 Add up your weekly income, ignoring any types of income that are not taken into account.

3 Check the 'appropriate amount' for someone in your circumstances – this is the minimum level of income you are expected to live on.

4 Work out the difference between your income and the appropriate amount to see if you are entitled to Guarantee Credit.

5 If you (or your partner if you have one) are aged 65 or over, check if you are entitled to Savings Credit by working out your 'qualifying income' and following the calculation set out below.

1 Your savings

Throughout this book the term 'savings' is used to cover savings, capital, investments and property. Savings are assessed in the same way for both the Guarantee Credit and the Savings Credit. Some forms of savings, including your home if you own it, are not taken into account, as explained below.

For Pension Credit, up to £10,000 savings, and any income you receive from these savings, is ignored. For a couple, savings are added together, but the limit is the same. There is no upper savings limit for Pension Credit, but any savings of £10,000 or over will be counted as £1 a week 'assumed income' for every £500 (or part of £500) over £10,000. For example, if you have £11,200, this will be counted as a weekly income of £3 a week, while savings of £13,600 will be assessed as an income of £8 a week.

Savings are normally valued at their current market or surrender value. If there are expenses involved in selling them, 10% will be deducted. Most forms of savings and capital will be taken into account, including:

- cash;
- bank and building society accounts (including current accounts that do not pay interest);
- National Savings accounts and certificates (valued according to rules that The Pension Service will explain);
- premium bonds;
- income bonds;
- stocks and shares;
- property (other than your home); and
- a share of any savings you own jointly with other people – these will normally be divided equally by the number of joint owners to calculate your share (get advice if you need to value your share of a jointly owned property).

Some types of savings will be ignored, including:

- the value of your home if you own it and are living there;
- the surrender value of a life assurance policy (although, if a policy is cashed in, the money you receive will normally be counted);
- arrears of certain benefits, such as Attendance Allowance (AA), Disability Living Allowance (DLA) or

Income Support, are normally ignored for 52 weeks from the date you receive them (or if the arrears are £5,000 or over and due to an official error, they may be able to be ignored for as long as you are getting Pension Credit);

- a lump-sum payment received because you put off claiming your State Pension for 52 weeks or more (see pages 28–34);
- your personal possessions; and
- the £10,000 ex-gratia payment for Far Eastern Prisoners of War (see page 126).

There are also other forms of savings not listed here that are ignored, and there are circumstances when property or savings will not be taken into account for a certain period.

If your State Pension or other social security benefits are paid into your bank account, they should not be counted as your capital until their payment period has expired. For example, if you receive AA paid into your account every four weeks, the value of the four weeks' payment should be deducted from the amount treated as capital.

FOR MORE INFORMATION, see the Department for Work and Pensions (DWP) guide to Pension Credit, which is available only on the Direct Gov website (www.direct.gov.uk).

Deprivation of capital (notional capital)   If you 'deprive' yourself of savings in order to get benefit or to increase the amount of benefit, you will be treated as still having those savings. This is known as 'notional capital'. This might occur if you give money to your family or buy expensive items in order to gain benefit. However, you will not be assessed as having notional capital if you have paid off debts or if your spending was 'reasonable' in your circumstances. You should seek advice if you are refused benefit because of notional capital.

2 Your income

This section explains how your income is assessed for the Guarantee Credit. The main types of income that are counted and the main types of income, or parts of income, that are ignored are listed below. If you have any income from other sources, you will need to check whether or not it is included. Income is assessed after tax and NI contributions have been paid. (If you receive income without tax deducted but are due to pay tax on this at a later date, get advice.) For a couple, the income of both partners is added together.

Income that is taken into account includes:

- State Pensions;
- occupational and personal pensions;
- income from annuities;
- most social security benefits (but see below for some exceptions);
- earnings (but see below for amounts ignored);
- Working Tax Credit;
- income from boarders or sub-tenants (but see below for parts ignored);
- regular payments from equity release schemes;
- maintenance payments for you or your partner from a spouse or former spouse;
  and
- assumed income from savings over £10,000.

Income that will be fully ignored includes:

- Housing Benefit and Council Tax Benefit;
- Attendance Allowance;
- Disability Living Allowance;
- Social Fund payments;
- child maintenance payments;

- actual interest or income from savings or capital (interest is not counted as income, but once it is paid into an account it will be counted as part of your savings);
- the special War Widow's Pension for 'pre-1973 widows', which is now £78.48 (in addition to the £10 of a War Widow's Pension outlined below); and
- voluntary or charitable payments – for example, money given to you by a charity, family or friends.

The following are examples of parts of weekly income that will also be ignored:

- £5 of your earnings if you work and are single;
- £10 of your or your partner's earnings from work (if you both work, the maximum is still £10);
- £20 of earnings if you work and you are a carer receiving the carer addition or in certain circumstances when you or your partner is disabled (instead of the £5 or £10 listed above);
- £10 of a War Widow/Widower's Pension or War Disablement Pension; and
- £20 of any payment from a sub-tenant or boarder and, in the case of a boarder, half of any payment over £20.

Add up your total weekly income, including assumed income from savings over £10,000 but not including any income that is ignored, to give the weekly income used to work out your Guarantee Credit.

Qualifying income for Savings Credit

For Savings Credit, only 'qualifying income' is counted. This is the same as the income used to assess Guarantee Credit but with the following types of income deducted:

- Incapacity Benefit;
- Severe Disablement Allowance;

- contribution-based ESA;
- contribution-based JSA;
- Working Tax Credit; and
- maintenance payments for you or your partner from a spouse or former spouse.

Most older people tend not to have these sources of income, so all their assessed income is likely to be qualifying income. When this is the case, the same figure is used to work out both the Guarantee and the Savings Credit. However, if you do have one or more of the types of non-qualifying income outlined above (such as ESA), remember that this affects the way that your Savings Credit is worked out.

3 The 'appropriate amount'

This is the minimum amount of income that someone is considered to need for their day-to-day living expenses. It is officially called the 'appropriate minimum guarantee' but is often described as the 'appropriate amount', which is the term used in this book.

If your income is below the appropriate amount for someone in your circumstances, you will receive the Guarantee Credit to bring your income up to this level. For many people a 'standard amount' will apply (officially called the 'standard minimum guarantee') but the appropriate amount can include additional amounts for severe disability, for carers and for certain housing costs. It is possible to receive both the carer and the severe disability addition – for example, a disabled couple who provide a substantial amount of care for each other could receive both.

The standard appropriate amounts are:

Single person	£132.60
Couple	£202.40

Additional amount for severe disability/severe disability premium Within Pension Credit your standard minimum amount can be increased if you fulfil the conditions described below. For Housing Benefit and Council Tax Benefit it is called the 'severe disability premium', but the rates and rules are the same. The rates are:

Single person	£53.65
Couple, one person qualifying	£53.65
Couple, both qualifying	£107.30

You qualify if:

- you receive AA or the middle or highest level of the care component of DLA;
- you 'live alone' (but see below for the exceptions to this); and
- no one receives Carer's Allowance (which used to be called Invalid Care Allowance) for looking after you.

If you have a partner and you receive AA (or the middle or highest level of the care component of DLA), you will not normally be able to receive this addition because you will not be counted as 'living alone'. However, you can receive it if:

- your partner also gets AA (or the middle or highest level of the care component of DLA), or they are registered blind; and
- no one receives Carer's Allowance for looking after you; and
- you 'live alone'; in other words, there is no one else living with you and your partner other than a person who is not taken into account, as described below.

If your partner also receives AA (or the middle or highest level of the care component of DLA) and neither of you has a carer receiving Carer's Allowance, you will receive the double rate.

Living alone You will still be counted as living alone in some circumstances when you live with other people. For example, you can still get this addition if there is someone else in your household who also gets AA (or the middle or highest level of the care component of DLA), or someone who is registered blind, or a paid helper supplied by a charity, or in some cases where you are a joint tenant or joint owner and share the housing costs. If you are not sure if you qualify, seek further advice as the rules can be complicated.

Additional amount for carers/carer premium Within Pension Credit a carer supplement can be added to your supplement standard amount if you fulfil the conditions described below. For Housing Benefit and Council Tax Benefit it is called the 'carer premium', but the rates and rules are the same.

The rates are:

Single person	£30.05
Couple, one person qualifying	£30.05
Couple, both qualifying	£60.10

This addition is available to carers who are receiving Carer's Allowance (see pages 110–115). It is also given to people who have applied for Carer's Allowance and fulfil all the conditions but cannot receive it because they are getting another benefit instead. There is no upper age limit for applying for Carer's Allowance.

For example, if you are receiving a State Pension of £97.65 a week, you cannot be paid Carer's Allowance as well. If you apply for Carer's Allowance, you will receive a letter saying that you are entitled to Carer's Allowance but it cannot be paid. However, when you show this letter to The Pension Service (for Pension Credit) or the council (for Housing Benefit and Council Tax Benefit) they will award you the carer's addition or premium.

The carer addition/premium continues to be paid for eight weeks after the person you care for dies, or you cease being a carer for some other reason.

Effect on the disabled person's benefits If the person you care for receives the severe disability addition/premium (see above), and you are paid Carer's Allowance, they will lose the addition/premium worth £53.65 when you receive your first payment of Carer's Allowance. However, they will only lose the addition/premium if you are actually paid an amount of Carer's Allowance. They will not lose it if you are entitled to Carer's Allowance, but it cannot be paid because you are receiving a State Pension or another benefit. If you are not sure whether to claim Carer's Allowance or what the effect might be on the other person's benefit, get advice first.

4 Calculating your Guarantee Credit

Once you have worked out your appropriate amount – in other words, the standard amount of £132.60 a week for a single person or £202.40 a week for a couple, plus any additional amounts because you are a carer, severely disabled or have eligible housing costs (see pages 59–62) – compare this figure with your income.

If your income (including assumed income from savings) is less than your appropriate amount, you will receive Guarantee Credit to bring your income up to this level. If you (or your partner) are 65 or over and your qualifying income is more than the 'Savings Credit threshold' – £98.40 a week for a single person, £157.25 for a couple – you will also receive Savings Credit.

If your income is more than your appropriate amount, you will not get Guarantee Credit. You may still be entitled to Housing Benefit and/or Council Tax Benefit and, if you or your partner are aged 65 or over, to Savings Credit.

Example

Rose is aged 76, and lives alone in a council flat. Her income is the State Pension of £97.65 a week and an occupational pension of £10. She has savings of £950.

Rose adds up her income

State Pension	£97.65
Occupational pension	£10.00
Total	£107.65

Her appropriate amount is the standard amount for a single person (£132.60).

Rose's income of £107.65 a week is less than her appropriate amount of £132.60. The difference is £24.95. This is how much Guarantee Credit she will get on top of her State Pension.

Rose is also entitled to some Savings Credit (see page 65) and to Housing Benefit and Council Tax Benefit to cover all her rent and Council Tax.

Example

Bill and Mary are a married couple both aged 70. Their joint State Pensions come to £154.70 and Bill gets a pension of £50.10 a week from his old job. They live in their own home and they have savings of £17,010.

Bill and Mary add up their income

State Pension	£154.70
Occupational pension	£50.10
Weekly assumed income from savings	£15.00
Total	£219.80

Their appropriate amount is the standard amount for a couple (£202.40).

Their income of £219.80 is more than their appropriate amount of £202.40, so they do not qualify for Guarantee

Credit. However, they will be entitled to Savings Credit (see pages 65–66) and, depending on the level of their Council Tax, they might be entitled to some Council Tax Benefit.

Example

Andrew is 80 and lives alone in his own home. His State Pension (basic and additional) is £100.95 and he has an occupational pension of £75.00 a week. His savings are less than £10,000. In May 2009 he applied for Pension Credit but was turned down because his income was too high, although he received some Council Tax Benefit. In October 2009 he had a stroke. He now has difficulty getting dressed and washed but has been able to continue to live on his own with support. No one receives Carer's Allowance for looking after him. His local Age UK/Age Concern* helped him claim AA and reapply for Pension Credit.

Andrew's income, ignoring AA

State Pension	£100.95
Occupational pension	£75.00
Total	£175.95

Andrew's appropriate amount

Standard amount	£132.60
Severe disability addition	£53.65
Total	£186.25

His income is £10.30 less than his appropriate amount, so he receives £10.30 Guarantee Credit. He can now also receive the maximum amount of Savings Credit (£20.52) and Council Tax Benefit to cover all his Council Tax.

Help with housing costs

In addition to the standard amount and any additions if you are a carer or severely disabled, your Pension Credit

*Many local Age Concerns are changing their name to Age UK.

appropriate amount can include an additional sum for certain housing costs if you own your property. If you are a tenant, your rent and service charges can be covered by Housing Benefit.

Some of the housing costs that can be included are:

- mortgage interest;
- interest on a loan for certain repairs or improvements;
- ground rent; and
- certain service charges, but funding for support services comes through the 'Supporting People' scheme (in Scotland, this is known as 'Housing Support') – see page 135).

The maximum loan or mortgage that you can receive interest on is £100,000, or up to £200,000 if you were receiving JSA, ESA or Income Support before receiving Pension Credit. You may not receive interest on the full amount if your housing costs are considered too high taking into account your situation (for example, if the property is considered too large). Payment is only made towards the eligible mortgage interest and does not cover any payments towards arrears, capital or endowment policies. You will have to meet any shortfall in payments if your lender's interest rate is higher than the DWP's Standard Rate, which is used to calculate eligible mortgage interest payments. The housing costs element of Pension Credit is generally paid direct to your lender, provided they are participating in the Mortgage Interest Direct Scheme.

If you are receiving Pension Credit (or other income-related benefits such as Income Support, income-based JSA or income-related ESA) or have been receiving any of these within the previous 26 weeks, you may only receive help towards any new housing costs in very limited circumstances. You should seek advice if you are considering taking out a new loan while receiving an income-related benefit.

Deductions for people living in your home

The help provided towards your housing costs may be reduced if there is someone else living in your home apart from your partner or a dependent child. This is because people such as adult sons and daughters (often called 'non-dependants') are expected to contribute to housing costs. Deductions are made according to the age, circumstances and gross income of the non-dependant. However, no reduction will be made if you or your partner is blind, or you or your partner receives AA or the care component of DLA.

If you are 65 or over, changes due to non-dependants that would reduce your benefit should not apply until 26 weeks after the change of circumstances.

In certain other circumstances a non-dependant deduction will not apply. There are no deductions if the person living with you:

- is a full-time student and you or your partner has reached age 65;
- is a boarder or a full-time student (but deductions may be made in the summer vacation if the student is working);
- is receiving Pension Credit;
- is in receipt of income-related ESA but has not yet been awarded a work-related or support component;
- is under 25 and receiving Income Support or income-based JSA;
- is in receipt of a training allowance;
- normally lives elsewhere;
- normally shares your home but is in prison;
- has been in hospital for 52 weeks or more; or
- has had a deduction applied in respect of them from the householder's Housing Benefit.

The level of the deduction will depend on the age, circumstances and gross weekly income of the non-dependant. For example, if the person living with you is aged 18 or over and works 16 hours a week or more, the following deductions will be made:

Gross income of non-dependant	Weekly deduction
under £120.00	£7.40
£120.00 to £177.99	£17.00
£178.00 to £230.99	£23.35
£231.00 to £305.99	£38.20
£306.00 to £381.99	£43.50
£382.00 or more	£47.75

For others aged 18 or over, the deduction will be £7.40. If there is a couple living with you, only one deduction will be made.

Example

Marie is aged 64 and has a mortgage. Her mortgage interest is assessed as £30 a week, so her appropriate amount is worked out in the following way:

Standard amount	£132.60
Weekly mortgage interest	£30.00
Total	£162.60

Her daughter, who is 35, and earns £190 a week, comes to live with her. There will therefore be a deduction of £23.35 from the amount allowed for mortgage interest. Marie's total Pension Credit appropriate amount will then be reduced to £139.25. This means that she will receive Guarantee Credit if her total assessed income is less than this amount. She is under 65 and so is not entitled to Savings Credit.

5 Calculating your Savings Credit

If you (or your partner if you have one) are aged 65 or over, you may be entitled to Savings Credit, either in addition to Guarantee Credit or on its own. The maximum amount of Savings Credit you can receive is £20.52 for a single person or £27.09 for a couple. This section outlines how the Savings Credit is worked out and gives some examples. However, the calculation is quite complicated and the examples do not cover all circumstances. If you are not sure whether you qualify, you may want to apply anyway. Alternatively, The Pension Service or a local advice agency may be able to give you an idea of any possible entitlement, or, if you have access to the internet, you could look at the Pension Credit calculator provided by The Pension Service on the Direct Gov website (www.direct.gov.uk).

As a guide, if you are single and your appropriate amount is the standard amount of £132.60, you are likely to be entitled to Savings Credit if your weekly qualifying income is more than £98.40 and less than around £184.00. For a couple with a standard amount of £202.40, you will be likely to qualify if your weekly qualifying income is more than £157.25 and less than around £270.00. The closer your income is to these upper amounts the less Savings Credit you will receive.

If your appropriate amount is more than the standard amounts – because you get an addition for severe disability, caring or housing costs – you may get Savings Credit if your income is higher than £184.00 (single person) or £270.00 (couple).

To calculate your Savings Credit you need to know the following things:

1 Your 'income'. This is the income used to calculate Guarantee Credit – in other words, your total income including assumed income from savings but not

including types of income that are ignored, such as AA.

2 Your 'qualifying income'. This is your income as explained above minus any Incapacity Benefit, Severe Disablement Allowance, contribution-based ESA, contribution-based JSA, Working Tax Credit and maintenance payments for you or your partner from a spouse or former spouse.

3 Your appropriate amount, as explained above.

4 The 'Savings Credit threshold', which is £98.40 for a single person and £157.25 for a couple.

5 The maximum amount of Savings Credit you can receive, which is £20.52 for a single person or £27.09 for a couple.

Standard appropriate amount   The information in this section explains how to calculate your Savings Credit if your appropriate amount is the standard amount of £132.60 (single person) or £202.40 (couple). If your qualifying income is below £98.40 (single person) or £157.25 (couple), you will not be entitled to Savings Credit – otherwise one of paragraphs (a), (b) or (c) will apply to you. The examples in paragraph (a) will be entitled to both Guarantee Credit and Savings Credit, those in paragraphs (b) and (c), below, will be entitled to Savings Credit only.

a) **If your income is less than your appropriate amount and your qualifying income is above £98.40 (single person) or £157.25 (couple), you will be entitled to Savings Credit.**

Your Savings Credit will be 60% of the difference between your qualifying income and £98.40 if you are single or £157.25 if you have a partner, up to the maximum amounts. (Another way of saying this is that you will receive 60p for every £1 of qualifying income you have over the threshold up to the maximum amount.)

Example

In the example on page 58, **Rose** has a basic State Pension of £97.65 and an occupational pension of £10 a week. Her Savings Credit will be worked out like this:

Qualifying income	£107.65
Difference between income of £107.65 and savings threshold of £98.40	£9.25
Savings credit is 60% of £9.25 (the difference)	£5.55

Rose will receive £5.55 Savings Credit in addition to her £24.95 Guarantee Credit and her pensions of £107.65, making her total income £138.15.

b) **If your qualifying income is exactly £132.60 (single person) or £202.40 (couple), you will normally receive the maximum Savings Credit,** which is £20.52 for a single person and £27.09 for a couple. (If you have some non-qualifying income, you will receive less Savings Credit.)

c) **If all your income is qualifying income and it is more than £132.60 (single person) or £202.40 (couple), you will receive Savings Credit if your income is less than a certain amount,** which is around £184.00 for a single person and £270.00 for a couple. The closer your income is to these levels the less Savings Credit you will receive. The maximum Savings Credit of £20.52 for a single person, and £27.09 for a couple, will be reduced by 40% of the difference between your income and £132.60 (single person) or £202.40 (couple). (Another way of saying this is that the maximum Savings Credit is reduced by 40p for every £1 of income you have above these levels.)

Example

In the example on page 58, **Bill and Mary** cannot get Guarantee Credit because their income of £219.80 is more than £202.40 (their appropriate amount). Their Savings Credit is worked out like this:

Qualifying income	£219.80
Difference between their income and £202.40	£17.40
40% of this difference	£6.96
Their Savings Credit is the maximum Savings Credit of £27.09 minus £6.96 (40% of the difference)	£20.13

Appropriate amount above the standard amount If you receive an addition for severe disability, caring or housing costs (like Andrew in the example on page 59), you can receive Savings Credit at higher levels of income. (Examples are not given here but are included in the Age UK factsheet on Pension Credit.) It is worked out like this:

- If all your income is qualifying income and it is more than £98.40 (single person) or £157.25 (couple) but less than your appropriate amount, your Savings Credit will be 60% of the difference between your income and £98.40 (single person) or £157.25 (couple) up to the maximum amount of Savings Credit of £20.52 (single person) or £27.09 (couple).

- If all your income is qualifying income and it is the same as or more than the standard amount (£132.60 single person, £202.40 couple) but less than your appropriate amount, you will receive the maximum Savings Credit.

- If all your income is qualifying income and it is more than your appropriate amount, the maximum Savings Credit of £20.52 (single person) or £27.09 (couple) is reduced by 40% of the difference between your income and your appropriate amount. If the 40% is more than the maximum, you will not receive Savings Credit.

If you have non-qualifying income If you or your partner receives non-qualifying income, such as Incapacity Benefit or ESA, you may still receive Savings Credit as long as you have qualifying income over the Savings Credit threshold (£98.40 for a single person, £157.25 for a couple). However, the calculation is done a little differently. Contact The Pension Service or an advice agency if you need more information about this, or look at the example in the Pension Service technical guide for Pension Credit, which is available on the Direct Gov website (www.direct.gov.uk).

Pension Credit for people in different circumstances

Living in someone else's home   If you live in someone else's home as a member of their household – for example, with your son or daughter – Pension Credit will be worked out in the normal way.

Boarders and hostel dwellers   If you are living in a hotel, guest-house or hostel, or in board and lodgings, Pension Credit will be worked out in the normal way. You can claim Housing Benefit towards the rental element of your charges and some services. You will have to pay for meals, fuel and other items that are not covered by Housing Benefit from your weekly Pension Credit.

If you go into hospital   If you go into hospital, your Pension Credit can normally continue to be paid however long you are there and the Pension Credit standard minimum amount is not affected. However, if you receive a severe disability addition or carer addition, you may lose it, as these additions are linked to benefits, such as AA (see page 98) and Carer's Allowance, which can be affected by a hospital stay. This will reduce your Pension Credit or in some cases it may stop because without the addition you may no longer qualify for the benefit.

If you are single and have been in hospital over 52 weeks, your Pension Credit will normally remain the same unless you are no longer treated as being responsible for housing costs.

If you are a member of a couple and one of you is in hospital for over 52 weeks, you may both be treated as single for Pension Credit purposes.

If you go abroad   If you go abroad for a temporary stay, Pension Credit can be paid for up to 13 weeks. If you are planning to go abroad, contact The Pension Service to find out more about your position.

Care homes   Pension Credit for people in care homes is generally calculated as described here, but see pages 136–147 for the differences.

How to claim Pension Credit

You can claim Pension Credit in a number of ways. There is a special Pension Credit application line on 0800 99 1234 (free call). Staff will help you apply over the phone and will let you know what happens next, or if you prefer you can ask to be sent a form to be filled in. If English is not your first language, you (or someone on your behalf) can ring and arrangements will be made for an interpreter. You can also write for a claim form or obtain it from the Direct Gov website (www.direct.gov.uk). If you would like to have face-to-face help with the form, contact a local advice agency or the local Pension Service.

You may need to provide information to support your claim, such as details of your savings and private pensions. The Pension Service is encouraging people to take up their entitlement to Pension Credit, so it may contact you to ask if you would like more information or to make an application.

Backdating   Pension Credit can be backdated for up to three months, as long as you have fulfilled the conditions throughout that time.

Changes of circumstances and reassessments

When you are awarded Pension Credit you may be told that an 'assessed income period' has been set. This will mean that for the time stated (normally a period of up to five years) you will not need to report changes in your 'retirement provision'. By retirement provision The Pension Service means income from sources such as pensions, annuities, regular payments from an equity-release scheme, and savings. Adjustments will be made automatically for regular increases, such as an annual increase in your State or private pension if this happens. If you have a private pension, you will be asked if and how it is increased when you apply.

You will not need to tell The Pension Service about changes such as an increase in your savings. However, if your income from these sources goes down, you can contact The Pension Service, which will reassess your benefit and may increase the amount of Pension Credit. You still need to report other changes in circumstances, such as getting married, moving house, a change in earnings, or starting to receive certain social security benefits.

An assessed income period will not be set if you (or your partner) are not aged 65 or over. Even if you are over 65, you may not have an assessed income period in some circumstances; for example, if your situation is expected to change in the next year. Sometimes a period of less than five years is set. At the end of an assessed income period your Pension Credit will be reassessed.

People aged 75 or over are normally given an assessed income period that lasts indefinitely, and those whose assessed income period runs out after the age of 80 will not usually need to be reassessed. However, the indefinite assessed income period will not apply to someone aged 75 and over if their circumstances are expected to change soon, even if they are 80 or over. There are some changes that will bring an assessed income period to an end (see above).

If you are not given an assessed income period, you will need to report any changes in circumstances that may affect your benefit. When Pension Credit is awarded you will be given information about what changes in circumstances you need to report.

If you disagree with a decision

If you disagree with a decision that has been made about your Pension Credit, you can ask for the decision to be revised, or appeal against the decision (see pages 42–43). You also have the right to ask for more detailed information about why a decision was made.

FOR MORE INFORMATION, see the Age UK factsheet on Pension Credit, which is available from Age UK Advice on 0800 169 65 65, and Pension Service leaflet PC1L Pension Credit *or the more detailed guide PC10S.*

Housing benefit and council tax benefit

Housing Benefit is a social security benefit that provides help with rent, with certain service charges and, in Northern Ireland, with general rates. People who live in Northern Ireland and require information about rate rebates or the new Rate Relief Scheme should contact Age NI at the address on page 224.

Council Tax Benefit is a social security benefit that provides help in reducing your Council Tax. See also 'Help with the Council Tax' on pages 174–176, which gives information about other ways your Council Tax bill may be reduced that are not related to your income or savings. The information here applies only to people over Pension Credit qualifying age. The rules are different for younger people, so if you are under Pension Credit qualifying age (see the box at the beginning of this chapter), contact your council or a local advice agency for more information.

Housing Benefit and Council Tax Benefit are based on your income and savings. In general, you must have no more than £16,000 in savings, although the limit does not apply to people receiving the Guarantee Credit part of the Pension Credit or the second adult rebate within the Council Tax Benefit system. You must also be 'habitually resident' in the UK, and not excluded from claiming because of your immigration status. Housing Benefit and Council Tax Benefit are not taxable.

If you have a partner, the amount of benefit you get will be worked out on your combined savings and income. A 'partner' is the person you are married to or living with as if you are married, or your civil partner or the person you are living with as if you are civil partners. If you live with someone who is not your partner – such as a friend or a brother or sister – you are assessed separately and both of you can apply for help with your housing costs or Council Tax.

Who qualifies for Housing Benefit?

You may get Housing Benefit if you are responsible for paying rent and you fulfil the conditions outlined above.

Housing Benefit is available to council, housing association and private tenants and to people in the following circumstances:

- Boarders and people living in hostels may get Housing Benefit for the accommodation part of their charges.
- People living in a houseboat may get Housing Benefit for the mooring charges even if they own the houseboat.
- People living in a caravan or mobile home may get help with the site charges even if they own the caravan or mobile home.
- Joint tenants may receive Housing Benefit towards the part of the costs for which they are responsible.
- People living with a landlord who is a close relative may claim Housing Benefit if they live separately in

self-contained accommodation. However, they cannot claim benefit if they live in the same dwelling, or if it is not a 'commercial arrangement'. Get advice if you are unsure about your position.

Who qualifies for Council Tax Benefit?

There are two types of Council Tax Benefit – 'main Council Tax Benefit' and 'second adult rebate'. If you are responsible for paying the Council Tax, you may be able to receive main Council Tax Benefit provided that you fulfil the conditions outlined above. If you are jointly responsible for a bill with someone other than your partner, you can apply for help with your share of the tax.

The second adult rebate may be available to some people, regardless of their income and savings, who have one or more people with low incomes living with them. This is covered on page 86, while the rest of this section covers the main benefit scheme.

How to work out your benefit

Housing Benefit and Council Tax Benefit are worked out using similar calculations. The rules outlined below apply to both benefits unless stated otherwise. The rules for working out Housing Benefit, Council Tax Benefit and Pension Credit are broadly similar, but there are some differences.

To work out how much benefit you will get, take the following steps, which are then explained in detail below:

1 Calculate the maximum weekly rent and Council Tax for which you can get benefit.
2 Deduct an amount for any non-dependants living in your home.
3 Add up the value of your savings, but note that certain types of savings are ignored.

4 Add up your weekly income, but note that certain kinds of income are ignored.

5 Work out the amount the Government says you need to live on, called the 'applicable amount'.

6 Calculate your benefit according to the formula explained below.

7 For Housing Benefit, check that the benefit is above the minimum amount payable, which is 50p a week. There is no minimum payment for Council Tax Benefit.

If you are receiving Pension Credit Guarantee Credit, you do not need to work out your savings, income and applicable amount, as you will receive the maximum eligible benefit minus any deductions for non-dependants.

1 Your rent and Council Tax

For Housing Benefit purposes, rent is the payment made to occupy your home. It also covers certain service charges – for example, for furniture, cleaning communal areas, entry phones and rubbish removal. Since April 2003 other support services, such as wardens and community alarms, are not eligible for help but may be funded separately through a system called 'Supporting People'. (In Scotland, this is known as 'Housing Support'.) Local authorities receive a grant for funding support services, including those provided by wardens in retirement (sheltered) housing. (See page 135 for how you get help with your support services.)

The Local Housing Allowance (LHA) method of working out Housing Benefit was introduced in April 2008 for all new tenants renting accommodation from a private landlord. It also affects tenants already getting Housing Benefit who move into accommodation rented from a private landlord. If you live in council accommodation or social housing (for example, you rent from a housing association), the LHA will not affect you. With LHA, the rent on which your benefit is based will initially depend on who lives with you and the area where you live, rather than necessarily the actual rent your landlord charges. You can check how much LHA would be in your area by asking your council or going to the Direct Gov website (www.direct.gov.uk) and searching for 'local housing allowance'.

You cannot get benefit for water rates and sewerage charges. Homeowners cannot get Housing Benefit; however, you may get help with mortgage interest payments and certain other housing costs from Pension Credit, Income Support, income-related ESA or income-based JSA.

If you are a council or housing association tenant, the maximum Housing Benefit you can get is 100% of your assessed rent, including the service charges described above.

High rents   If you have been receiving Housing Benefit as a private tenant and you are not covered by the LHA rules, your benefit may have been restricted under older rules. This might have happened if the local authority decided that your rent was too high or your accommodation was larger than you needed (taking into account your circumstances) or that the rent has increased unreasonably while you have been getting Housing Benefit.

Local authorities can make 'discretionary housing payments' if they decide that you need further help with a shortfall in meeting your rent or Council Tax. So, if your benefit is restricted, you may want to apply for help under this scheme.

If you want to challenge a decision about your benefit or to ask the local authority to use its discretion, it is a good idea to get advice from a local advice agency. The rules on rent restrictions are complicated and are covered only briefly here. If you need more information, contact Age UK or consult a book such as the *Welfare Benefits and Tax Credits Handbook* (see page 211).

Council Tax The maximum Council Tax Benefit you can get is 100% of your bill.

Council Tax Benefit is based on the amount you are asked to pay after any 'discounts' or 'reductions' (see pages 174–176) have been given. For example, if you live alone, you will receive a 25% discount on your bill, and your benefit will be worked out after this has been deducted.

Note that the calculations in this section are all done on a weekly basis. So if you pay your Council Tax in 10 monthly instalments, you will first have to work out how much this would be per week over the whole year.

Heating charges Some people have a charge for heating included in their rent. You cannot get Housing Benefit for heating and other fuel charges. If, for example, you pay £45 a week rent and £5 of that is for heating, you will only get a maximum of £40 Housing Benefit, as the charge for fuel will be deducted. If your weekly fuel charges are not stated as a separate amount, the council will deduct the amounts listed as follows:

Heating	£21.55
Hot water	£2.50
Cooking	£2.50
Lighting	£1.75
All fuel	£28.30

The amounts are lower if you occupy only one room.

2 Deductions for non-dependants living in your home

A deduction will normally be made from both your Housing Benefit and your Council Tax Benefit if you have someone else living with you who is neither your partner or a dependent child nor a joint tenant or joint owner. This is because people such as grown-up sons and daughters (called 'non-dependants') are expected to contribute to housing costs. However, no deduction will be made if you or your partner is blind or receive AA or the care component of DLA. There are also some types of non-dependant who do not give rise to a deduction – for example, full-time students during term time.

There will be no deduction from your Housing Benefit if the person who lives with you receives Pension Credit, or is under 25 and receives Income Support or income-based JSA, or is under 25 and receives income-related ESA that does not include a component. There will be a £7.40 deduction from your Housing Benefit for anyone else who is aged 18 or over and does not fall into any of the categories already mentioned.

If the person living with you is aged 18 or over, works 16 or more hours a week and has a gross income of at least £120 a week, the rates of deduction are as follows:

Housing Benefit

Gross income of non-dependant	Weekly deduction from Housing Benefit
under £120.00	£7.40
£120.00 to £177.99	£17.00
£178.00 to £230.99	£23.35
£231.00 to £305.99	£38.20
£306.00 to £381.99	£43.50
£382 or more	£47.75

Council Tax Benefit

Gross income of non-dependant	Weekly deduction from Council Tax Benefit
Less than £178.00	£2.30

£178.00 to £305.99	£4.60
£306.00 to £381.99	£5.80
£382 or more	£6.95

Deductions are made from your Council Tax Benefit for non-dependants aged over 18 who normally live with you. There are four levels of deduction. If the non-dependant is working less than 16 hours per week, the lowest deduction will apply. If the non-dependant is doing paid work for 16 hours or more a week, the level of deduction will depend on the non-dependant's gross weekly income.

For Council Tax Benefit there are some types of non-dependants who do not give rise to a deduction (such as full-time students). There is no deduction for a non-dependant receiving Pension Credit, Income Support, income-based JSA or income-related ESA, while for others aged 18 or over not covered above there will be a £2.30 deduction.

Only one deduction is made for a non-dependent couple living with you.

A deduction may be delayed for 26 weeks if you or your partner are aged 65 or over and a non-dependant moves into your home, or the non-dependant's circumstances change to increase the deduction.

3 Your savings

Throughout this book the term 'savings' is used to cover savings, capital, investments and property.

If your savings are more than £16,000, you cannot normally get Housing Benefit or the main Council Tax Benefit. However, if you are receiving the Guarantee Credit part of Pension Credit, there is no savings limit. For a couple, savings are added together, but the limit is the same. If you are over Pension Credit qualifying age, you can have up to £10,000 in savings without it affecting your benefit (people under this age can have up to £6,000 without affecting their benefit).

If you are over the Pension Credit qualifying age and not receiving Pension Credit Guarantee Credit and have savings of between £10,000 and £16,000, an income of £1 a week for every £500 (or part of £500) over £10,000 will be taken into account in working out your benefit. For example, if you have savings of £11,480, you will be treated as having an income of £3 a week. Savings of £14,750, will be treated as £10 a week. This is called 'tariff income'. Savings of £10,000 or less will not affect your benefit.

If you are under the qualifying age for Pension Credit and have savings of between £6,000 and £16,000, an income of £1 a week for every £250 (or part of £250) over £6,000 will be taken into account in working out your benefit. For example, if you have savings of £6,300, you will be treated as having an income of £2 per week.

Savings and capital are normally valued at their current market or surrender value. If there are expenses involved in selling them, 10% will be deducted. Most forms of savings and capital will be taken into account, including:

- cash;
- bank and building society accounts (including current accounts that do not pay interest);
- National Savings & Investments accounts and certificates (valued according to rules, which the local authority will explain);
- premium bonds;
- income bonds;
- stocks and shares;
- property (other than your home); and
- a share of any savings you own jointly with other people – these will normally be divided equally by the

number of joint owners to calculate your share (get advice if you need to value your share of jointly owned property).

Some types of savings will be ignored, including:

- the value of your home if you own it and are living there;
- the surrender value of a life assurance policy (although if a policy is cashed in, the money you receive will normally be counted);
- arrears of certain benefits, such as AA, DLA or Income Support, for 52 weeks from the date you receive them (or longer if the arrears are £5,000 or over and due to an official error);
- a lump-sum payment received because you put off claiming your State Pension;
- your personal possessions; and
- the £10,000 ex-gratia payment for Far Eastern Prisoners of War (see page 126).

There are also other forms of savings not listed here that are ignored, and there are circumstances when property or savings will not be taken into account for a certain period of time – contact the council or a local advice agency for more information.

Deprivation of capital (notional capital) If you 'deprive' yourself of savings in order to get benefit or to increase the amount of benefit, you will be treated as still having those savings. This is known as 'notional capital'. This might occur if you give money to your family or buy expensive items in order to gain benefit. However, you will not be assessed as having notional capital if you have paid off debts or if your spending was 'reasonable' in your circumstances. You should seek advice if you are refused benefit because of notional capital.

4 Your income

This section lists the main types of income that are counted and the type of income, or parts of income, that are ignored when working out Housing Benefit and Council Tax Benefit for people over the qualifying age for Pension Credit. If you have any income from other sources, you will need to check whether or not they are included. Income is assessed after tax and NI contributions have been paid. For a couple, the income of both partners is added together.

Income that is taken into account includes:

- State Pensions;
- occupational and personal pensions;
- the Savings Credit part of Pension Credit if you are not receiving the Guarantee Credit (if you receive Pension Credit Guarantee Credit, your other income or savings will not affect your Housing Benefit or Council Tax Benefit);
- income from annuities;
- most social security benefits (but see below for some exceptions);
- earnings (but see below for amounts ignored);
- Working Tax Credit;
- income from boarders or sub-tenants (but see below for parts ignored);
- regular payments from equity-release schemes;
- maintenance payments for you or your partner from a spouse or former spouse; and
- assumed income from savings over £10,000.

Income that will be fully ignored includes:

- Pension Credit Guarantee Credit;
- Attendance Allowance;

- Disability Living Allowance;
- child maintenance;
- actual interest or income from savings or capital (only assumed income will be counted, as explained above); interest is not counted as income but once it is paid into an account it will be counted as part of your savings;
- the special War Widow's Pension for 'pre-1973 widows', which is now £78.48 (in addition to the £10 of a War Widow/Widower's Pension outlined below); and
- voluntary or charitable payments – for example, money given to you by a charity, family or friends.

The following are examples of parts of weekly income that will also be ignored:

- £5 of your earnings if you work and are single;
- £10 of your or your partner's earnings from work;
- £20 of earnings if you work and you are a carer receiving the carer premium, or in certain circumstances when you or your partner is disabled (instead of the £5 or £10 listed above);
- £10 of a War Widow/Widower's Pension or War Disablement Pension (the local authority has the discretion to increase the amount from these pensions that is ignored when working out your benefit, but not all authorities operate such schemes: contact your local authority for more information); and
- £20 of any payment from a sub-tenant or boarder and, in the case of a boarder, half of any payment over £20.

To work out your benefit, decide what kinds of income will be ignored and add up the remainder (including tariff income for savings between £6,000 and £16,000).

5 Your applicable amount

This is the weekly amount that is compared with your income to calculate your Housing Benefit and Council Tax Benefit. If your income is higher than this, you may still get some help with rent and the Council Tax. The basic personal allowances for people who have reached the Pension Credit qualifying age are:

> *Single person aged under 65
> £132.60
>
> *Couple, one or both 60–64, both under 65
> £202.40
>
> Single person aged 65 or over
> £153.15
>
> Couple, one or both aged 65 or over
> £229.50
>
> *The personal allowances for people who have not yet attained the Pension Credit qualifying age are lower. For more information contact a local advice agency.

In addition to these basic amounts you may also be entitled to a severe disability premium or a carer premium (or sometimes both). The rules for these are the same as for the additions in Pension Credit and are described on pages 55–56.

For people under 65 the applicable amount is the same as the 'appropriate amount' in Pension Credit. For people aged 65 and over the amount is higher.

However, if you or your partner is not entitled to guarantee Pension Credit, any Savings Credit you receive will be taken into account in your Housing Benefit or Council Tax Benefit.

6 Calculating Housing Benefit and Council Tax Benefit

Once you have worked out your applicable amount, compare this figure with your income, including any tariff income from savings over £10,000. If your income is the same as, or less than your applicable amount, you will normally get all your rent and Council Tax paid (unless, for example, there are deductions for ineligible service charges, for other people living in your home or because your rent is considered too high). If you are not already receiving Pension Credit, you may be entitled to it, so you should consider applying.

If your income is more than your applicable amount, the maximum benefit you can get is reduced. You first work out the difference between your income and your applicable amount. The maximum Housing Benefit payable is reduced by 65% of this difference. The maximum Council Tax Benefit is reduced by 20% of the difference.

Another way of explaining the calculation is to say that your maximum Housing Benefit is reduced by 65p for every £1 that your income is more than your applicable amount. Your maximum Council Tax Benefit is reduced by 20p for every £1 that your income is more than your applicable amount.

Example

Julie is aged 64 and lives alone. Her income consists of a State Pension (basic and additional) of £100 a week. She has £2,000 in savings and pays £50 a week in rent and £14 a week in Council Tax (after the 25% discount because she lives alone).

The maximum Housing Benefit she can get is £50 a week (100% of her rent). The maximum Council Tax Benefit she can get is £14 a week (100% of her Council Tax). There are no deductions for non-dependants because she lives alone.

Her savings will not affect her benefit as they are less than £10,000. Julie's applicable amount is the standard personal allowance for someone aged under 65 (£132.60).

Her income is less than her applicable amount, so she will get the maximum Housing Benefit of £50 a week for rent and the maximum Council Tax Benefit of £14 a week. She will also qualify for Pension Credit Guarantee Credit and should make a claim.

Example

Amir and Samina are both aged 68 and live in a rented house. Amir receives AA and Samina cares for him. She applied for Carer's Allowance and although she satisfied the caring conditions she cannot be paid it because she is receiving a State Pension worth more than the allowance. However, this means that she has an 'underlying entitlement' to Carer's Allowance, so they qualify for the carer premium.

They pay £58 a week in rent. Their Council Tax is £16 a week. They have State Pensions of £160 a week between them, Amir's occupational pension of £90.00 a week, Pension Credit Savings Credit of £15.27 a week and savings of £15,700.

The maximum Housing Benefit they can get is £58. The maximum Council Tax Benefit they can get is £16. They have nobody else living with them, so there will be no deductions for non-dependants.

Amir and Samina add up their income

State Pension	£160.00
Occupational pension	£90.00
Tariff income (for savings over £10,000)	£12.00
Pension Credit Savings Credit	£15.27
Total	£277.27

They calculate their applicable amount

Personal allowance	£229.50
Carer premium	£30.05
Total	£259.55

Their income is more than their applicable amount, the difference being £17.72 (£277.27 – £259.55).

Their weekly benefit is worked out in the following way:

Rent

100% of rent	£58.00
Less 65% of difference (65% of £17.72)	£11.52
Housing Benefit (£65 – £11.52)	£46.48

Council Tax

100% of tax	£16.00
Less 20% of difference (20% of £17.72)	£3.55
Council Tax Benefit (£16 - £3.55)	£12.45

Total benefit is

Housing Benefit	£46.48
Council Tax Benefit	£12.45

Amir and Samina will have to pay £11.52 a week for rent and £3.55 towards the Council Tax.

Example

George and Anne are both 78 and own their home. Their Council Tax is £20 a week. Their weekly income consists of State Pensions of £154.70 a week, income from an annuity of £46, and £67.70 from an occupational pension. They also have £17,800 savings.

They have never claimed benefits before but were worried because they were having to use their savings to pay their Council Tax bill. They asked their local advice agency about Pension Credit. It was explained that at present they would not be entitled to Pension Credit but they were advised to claim Council Tax Benefit. The maximum Council Tax Benefit they can get is £20. They have nobody else living with them, so there will be no deductions for non-dependants.

George and Anne add up their income

State Pension	£154.70
Occupational pension	£67.70
Annuity income	£46.00
Tariff income from savings	£16.00
Total	£284.40

Their applicable amount is the basic personal allowance for a couple aged over 65 (£229.50).

Their income is £54.90 more than their applicable amount.

Their weekly benefit is worked out in the following way:

Council Tax

100% of tax	£20.00
Less 20% of difference (20% of £54.90)	£10.98
Council Tax Benefit	£9.02

George and Anne will receive £9.02 a week (£469.04 over the year) towards their Council Tax. If their granddaughter, who is aged 25 and earning £200 a week, comes to live with them, she will be counted as a 'non-dependant' and their benefit will be reduced by £4.60 a week.

Second adult rebate

If you are solely liable to pay the Council Tax, you might get a second adult rebate if one or more people with a low income live with you, regardless of the level of your savings and income. This will usually apply only to people who do not have a partner.

You may get a 25% rebate if you are responsible for the Council Tax and you have living with you one or more people receiving Pension Credit, Income Support, income-based JSA or income-related ESA. A 15% rebate is given if the person or people living with you have a joint gross income of less than £175.00; there is a 7.5% rebate if their income is between £175.00 and £227.99. In assessing the income of people living with you, no account is taken of AA, DLA or the income of anyone receiving Pension Credit, Income Support, income-based JSA or income-related ESA.

Example

Janice is a widow who owns her own home. Her son is living with her and receives income-based JSA. Her Council Tax bill for the year is £800. She is not entitled to the main Council Tax Benefit because she has £18,000 in savings. However, she applies for a rebate and receives the second adult rebate of 25% (£200) because her son receives income-based JSA.

Some people will be entitled to the main Council Tax Benefit and the second adult rebate. In this case the local authority will award you whichever benefit will give you the greater amount.

Only brief details have been given here as this system can be complicated, so contact the council or a local advice agency if you need further information.

Benefit for people in different circumstances

Absence from home   If you go into hospital on a temporary basis, you can continue to get Housing Benefit and Council Tax Benefit for up to 52 weeks (provided that you intend to return home). If you are temporarily away from home for other reasons, benefit will be paid for up to 13 weeks or up to 52 weeks, depending on the reason for your absence. Contact the council or a local advice agency if you need more information about this. You cannot get benefit if you sub-let your home while you are away.

Benefit for two homes   You can normally only get Housing Benefit for one home. However, there are some circumstances in which payments may be made for two homes. For example, you may qualify for benefit on two homes for up to four weeks if you have moved to a new home and it is reasonable that you could not avoid liability to make payments for both homes. Another example is where your move to a new home has been delayed because it was being adapted to meet disability needs. Entitlement to Housing Benefit for two homes is not automatic, so ask your local authority whether you qualify.

Council Tax Benefit is payable only for the home in which you normally live. It is not payable for second homes.

Discretionary housing payments   You can apply to the local authority for an extra payment towards your rent and Council Tax if you are having difficulty meeting your bills. Your local authority will tell you how to make a claim and you will be able to give reasons why you need additional support.

How to claim

If you are claiming Pension Credit,   you should also be asked if you want to apply for Housing Benefit and Council Tax Benefit; you will be given a short three-page form, which will mean that you do not need to give much of the same information to both The Pension Service and the local authority. If you are claiming Pension Credit over the phone, the staff there will fill in the Housing Benefit and Council Tax Benefit claim form for you at the same time. Since October 2008 The Pension Service has been able to forward all the information about your claim directly to the local authority so they can work out your Housing Benefit and Council Tax Benefit without your having to sign and return a form.

If you are not claiming Pension Credit,   you claim Housing Benefit and Council Tax Benefit directly from your local authority. Before the local authority can work out how much to pay, it may require evidence such as details of your income, savings and the amount of rent you pay.

If you are a couple, only one of you should claim for benefit – it does not matter if the bill is sent in joint names or to just one of you. Your benefit will be calculated on the basis of your combined income and savings.

Backdating Housing Benefit and Council Tax Benefit can be backdated for up to three months as long as you have satisfied the conditions during that time.

If your circumstances change If you are not receiving Pension Credit, you must report any changes that might affect your Housing Benefit or Council Tax Benefit to the local authority. If you are receiving Pension Credit, whether you need to tell the local authority about changes will depend on the nature of the change and which part of Pension Credit you are receiving. For example, if you are receiving Pension Credit Guarantee Credit, you will not need to report changes in your income and savings to the local authority. You may need to report these changes to The Pension Service, depending on whether or not you have an assessed income period (see pages 68–70).

If you are receiving the Savings Credit but not the Guarantee Credit, you must tell the local authority about some changes. These include an increase in your savings to over £16,000, regardless of whether or not you have a Pension Credit assessed income period.

Your local authority will tell you about when you need to let it know if your circumstances change. If you are unsure, contact the local authority to check; otherwise, you could have to repay money you have been overpaid or receive less benefit than you are entitled to.

Delays and administrative problems The local authority should let you know within 14 days of your claim whether you qualify for help (as long as you have provided any information and evidence needed). However, this sometimes takes much longer. If you are suffering hardship because the local authority has not yet worked out your claim for benefit or you are having problems with your benefit, contact a local advice agency or Citizens Advice for help.

How it is paid

For council tenants, Housing Benefit is usually paid by reducing the rent. If you are a private or housing association tenant, your Housing Benefit may be paid to you by cheque or into a bank account or direct to your landlord.

Most people will pay the Council Tax direct to their local authority, so when you claim benefit your bill will be reduced accordingly. Where this is not possible because, for example, you have already paid the whole bill, the local authority may send you a refund or credit your account.

Overpayment If you are paid too much benefit, this is known as an overpayment and in most circumstances the local authority can ask you to repay this money. However, an overpayment cannot normally be recovered if it was caused by an 'official error' and you could not reasonably be expected to have known you were being overpaid at the time. Even if the local authority can recover the benefit, it does have some discretion about whether to do so. It is a good idea to seek further advice if you are being asked to repay benefit.

If you disagree with a decision

If you disagree with a decision about your Housing Benefit or Council Tax Benefit, you can ask for the decision to be revised, or appeal to an independent tribunal (see pages 42–43).

THE SOCIAL FUND

The Social Fund provides lump-sum payments for expenses that are difficult to meet from low income. There are

Funeral Payments, which are described on pages 193–195, and Cold Weather Payments, which are explained on page 166. In addition there are Winter Fuel Payments, which are not related to income (see page 165). If you have other expenses – for example, if you need a cooker or bedding – you may get help from the discretionary Social Fund in the form of Community Care Grants, Budgeting Loans or Crisis Loans, which are covered in this section.

The payments described here are different from most other social security benefits in that they are discretionary, and Budgeting Loans and Crisis Loans have to be repaid. There is a limited budget for the discretionary Social Fund, which restricts the overall amount that can be awarded in grants and loans in any financial year. There is a legal framework for the system and Social Fund decision-makers have to follow legal rules called 'directions' and take account of guidance that helps them make decisions. For Community Care Grants and Crisis Loans they must consider all the individual circumstances of the people who apply and decide which applications can be met from the budget. Awards of Budgeting Loans are more 'fact-based', as explained below, rather than being wholly discretionary, but they must still be made from a fixed budget.

Community Care Grants

These are available to people receiving Pension Credit, Income Support, income-related ESA, income-based JSA, and to people who will be discharged from care within six weeks and are likely to receive these benefits on discharge. The grants do not have to be repaid. The amount of any savings you have over £1,000 (£500 for people under Pension Credit qualifying age) will be deducted from any grant awarded. For example, if you qualify for Pension Credit and have £1,100 savings and you need an item costing £300 you would only receive a grant for £200. If you are not sure whether you will get help, you have nothing to lose by applying. It is important to include all the relevant information (see below on 'How to apply').

Grants are available for certain purposes, including:

- help with moving out of institutional or residential care (for example, for a bed, a cooker, fuel connection or removal costs);
- help to enable you to remain living at home (for example, for minor house repairs, bedding and essential furniture or removal costs to more suitable accommodation);
- help to ease exceptional pressures on families (for example, caused by disability, chronic sickness or a breakdown in a relationship); and
- help with certain travel expenses (for example, for visiting someone who is ill or attending a relative's funeral).

FOR MORE INFORMATION, see Age UK factsheet The Social Fund, *Jobcentre Plus leaflet DWP1007* The Social Fund *or detailed guide SB16* A Guide to the Social Fund, *which is available only online from the DWP website (www.dwp.gov.uk).*

Budgeting Loans

These are available to people who have been receiving Pension Credit, Income Support, income-based JSA or income-related ESA for at least 26 weeks. They enable people to spread the cost of one-off expenses over a longer period. The loans, which are interest-free, have to be repaid, and the amount of any savings over £2,000 (£1,000 for people under Pension Credit qualifying age) will reduce the amount of the loan.

The applications for Budgeting Loans and Community Care Grants are separate. So consider whether you might qualify for a grant before applying for a Budgeting Loan. You may be able to get a Budgeting Loan for one of the following:

- furniture and household equipment;
- clothing and footwear;
- removal costs and/or rent in advance;
- home improvements, maintenance or home security measures;
- travel expenses;
- expenses associated with seeking or going back to work; or
- hire purchase (HP) and other debts (for expenses associated with the categories outlined).

In deciding whether you can be awarded a loan, the Social Fund decision-maker will look at whether you:

- have been receiving benefit for at least 26 weeks;
- are single, a couple or either single or a couple with children; and
- owe loans already to the Social Fund.

Crisis Loans

These interest-free loans are available to anyone (not just people receiving benefits such as Pension Credit) who needs something urgently in an emergency or as a result of a disaster (such as fire or flood). The Social Fund decision-maker will take into account any family savings or income available to you. You may be able to get a loan, provided that this is the only way of preventing serious damage or risk to your health or safety or that of a member of your family.

Repayment of loans

Budgeting or Crisis Loans will be awarded only if the officer thinks you will be able to repay them. Loan repayments will normally be deducted from your benefit and have to be repaid within 104 weeks. In special circumstances the repayment period may be extended further.

The repayment rates will be fixed after taking into account your income and your existing commitments. In the case of Crisis Loans, repayments will not normally begin until after the period of crisis is over.

If you take out a further loan from the Social Fund whilst still repaying an earlier loan, repayment of the further loan will not begin until the original loan has been repaid.

The repayment arrangements can be changed if you are having difficulty paying the original rate of repayment. If you are having difficulties, contact your Jobcentre Plus to discuss the level of repayment rate.

How to apply

To get application forms for a Community Care Grant or a Budgeting Loan, or to apply for a Crisis Loan, contact Jobcentre Plus by visiting the website (www.jobcentreplus.gov.uk) or by phone, using the number in your local phone book.

When applying for a Community Care Grant or Crisis Loan, give as much information as possible about your circumstances and why you need help (for example, health problems). If there is not enough room on the form, use a separate sheet.

A local advice agency or Citizens Advice may be able to help you with the application. You may also wish to include a letter of support from your GP or social worker.

If you are unhappy about a decision

Community Care Grants and loans from the Social Fund are discretionary payments. If you disagree with a decision, you cannot appeal to an appeal tribunal, but instead there is a special system of review. A request for a review must be made in writing and give reasons why you think the decision is wrong. You should make the request within 28 days of the decision. The first stage of review is at Jobcentre Plus and you may be offered an interview. This is usually done over the phone rather than in person. If you are still dissatisfied, you can take your case to the Independent Review Service where it will be considered by a Social Fund Inspector, who is independent of your local Jobcentre Plus office. A local advice agency may be able to help if you want to ask for a review.

FOR MORE INFORMATION, see Jobcentre Plus leaflet DWP1007 The Social Fund or detailed guide SB16, which is available only on the DWP website (www.dwp.gov.uk).

Disability Benefits and Paying for Care

This part of *Your Rights to Money Benefits* describes the main Department for Work and Pensions (DWP) benefits available to people who are ill or disabled and those who look after them.

Disability Living Allowance (DLA) and Attendance Allowance (AA) are the most important benefits for people with disabilities. They are intended to help with the extra costs associated with disability.

Carer's Allowance is paid to people who provide care for disabled people who receive the middle or highest-rate care component of DLA, AA or Constant Attendance Allowance (CAA) (see page 125).

Employment and Support Allowance (ESA) is the new benefit for people who are unable to work due to sickness or disability, although some people will continue to receive Incapacity Benefit or Severe Disablement Allowance (SDA).

There is also a section about paying for care – either in your own home or in a care home – which includes information about local authority charging procedures and financial support.

ATTENDANCE ALLOWANCE AND DISABILITY LIVING ALLOWANCE

AA and DLA are intended to provide help towards the extra costs arising from physical or mental disability. Which one you claim depends on your age.

To qualify for DLA you must need help with personal care or have difficulty walking and you must claim before your 65th birthday. If you are 65 or over and need help with personal care, you should claim AA instead.

This section covers first the conditions for AA and then the conditions for DLA; the third part gives information that applies to both allowances.

Attendance Allowance

This is a benefit for people aged 65 or over who need help with personal care, or need supervision by day or someone to watch over them by night, because of physical or mental disability. It does not depend on National Insurance (NI) contributions, is not affected by savings or income (other than CAA), and is paid on top of other benefits or pensions. AA is not taxable.

There are two weekly rates:

Higher rate	£71.40
Lower rate	£47.80

Who qualifies for Attendance Allowance?

To qualify for AA you must fulfil all the following conditions:

- you are aged 65 or older;
- you meet the day and/or night conditions described below;
- you must also normally have satisfied the disability conditions for at least six months, but there are

'special rules' for people who are terminally ill, as explained on pages 108–109.

You will receive the lower rate if you fulfil either the day or the night conditions. You will get the higher rate if you fulfil both day and night conditions. You can receive the allowance if you live alone or with other people and regardless of whether or not you receive any help from someone else – what matters is that you need help with personal care, supervision or watching over, not whether you are actually getting help. You do not have to spend the allowance on paying for care: it is up to you how you use it. However, your local authority may take it into account when assessing whether, and how much, you need to pay for any care services you have.

Day conditions   You may fulfil the day-time condition if you are so disabled that you require frequent help throughout the day with your normal 'bodily functions', such as eating, getting in or out of bed, going to the toilet or washing. 'Seeing' and 'hearing' are considered bodily functions. For example, if you are visually impaired and need someone to read your post, or if you are deaf and need help with communicating, this could help you satisfy the requirement for needing 'frequent help'. You may also fulfil the day-time condition if you need continual supervision throughout the day to avoid putting yourself or others in substantial danger, or if you need someone with you when you are on renal dialysis.

Night conditions   You may fulfil the night-time condition if you are so disabled that you require prolonged (generally periods of at least 20 minutes) or repeated (generally at least twice nightly) attention during the night to help you with your bodily functions – for example, going to the toilet and getting in and out of bed. You may also fulfil the night-time condition if another person needs to be awake for a prolonged period or at frequent intervals at night in order to watch over you to avoid putting yourself or others in substantial danger.

The next section covers the qualifying conditions for DLA. You should turn to pages 105–110 for information that covers both allowances, such as how to make a claim and what happens if you are away from home.

Disability Living Allowance

This benefit is for people who make a claim before the age of 65, and who, because of their physical or mental disability:

- need help with personal care, or need supervision by day, or need someone to watch over them at night; or
- are unable to walk, have great difficulty walking, or need someone with them when walking in unfamiliar places outdoors; or
- need help with both of these.

DLA does not depend on NI contributions, is not affected by savings or income (other than CAA or War Pensioners' Mobility Supplement) and is paid on top of other benefits or pensions. DLA is not taxable.

There are two parts to DLA: the 'care component', which is paid at one of three rates, and the 'mobility component', which has two different levels. The weekly rates are:

DLA care component

Highest rate	£71.40
Middle rate	£47.80
Lowest rate	£18.95

DLA mobility component

Higher rate	£49.85
Lower rate	£18.95

Who qualifies for DLA?   To qualify for DLA you *must* fulfil all the following conditions:

- you meet one or more of the care or mobility conditions described below;
- you are aged under 65 when you claim;
- you have also normally satisfied the disability conditions for at least three months, and are expected to satisfy them for at least the next six months, but there are 'special rules' for people who are terminally ill, as explained on pages 108–109.

Rules about your age   Although you must have become disabled, and made a claim, before the age of 65, once you are awarded DLA it will continue, without an age limit, as long as you satisfy either the care or the mobility conditions. If you are receiving the lowest or middle rate of the care component and your care needs change after you are 65, you may be able to qualify for a higher rate after six months. You cannot normally start to receive the lowest rate of the care component or any rate of the mobility component after the age of 65. However, you may be able to receive it if you are already getting one of the components and you can show that you met the conditions for the other component before the age of 65. Seek advice if you think that this may apply to you.

The care component   The care component of DLA is for people who need help with personal care, supervision or watching over because of physical or mental disability. It does not matter if you live alone or with other people, or whether or not you receive any help from someone else – what matters is that you need help with personal care, supervision or watching over, not whether you are actually getting help. You do not have to spend the allowance on paying for care: it is up to you how you use it. However, your local authority may take it into account when assessing whether, and how much, you need to pay for any care services you receive.

You will receive £18.95 if you fulfil one of the lowest-rate conditions.

Lowest-rate conditions

You may fulfil this condition if you need help with 'bodily functions' for a significant portion of the day. For example, you might need some help to get up in the morning and go to bed in the evening but manage alone for the rest of the day. You may also fulfil this condition if, as a result of your disability, you could not prepare a main cooked meal for yourself.

Middle and highest rate conditions

You will receive the middle rate if you fulfil either a day or a night condition. The highest rate is for those who fulfil both a day and a night condition.

Day conditions   You may fulfil the day-time condition if you are so disabled that you require frequent help throughout the day with your normal bodily functions, such as eating, getting in or out of bed, going to the toilet or washing. Seeing and hearing are bodily functions. For example, if you are visually impaired and need someone to read your post, or you are deaf and need help with communicating, this could help you satisfy the requirement for needing 'frequent help'. You may also fulfil the condition if you need continual supervision throughout the day to avoid putting yourself or others in substantial danger, or if you need someone with you when you are on renal dialysis.

Night conditions   You may fulfil the night-time condition if you are so disabled that you require prolonged (generally periods of at least 20 minutes) or repeated (generally at least twice nightly) attention during the night to help you with your bodily functions – for example, going to the toilet and getting in and out of bed. You may also fulfil this condition if another person needs to be awake for a prolonged period or at frequent intervals throughout the night to watch over you to avoid putting yourself or others in substantial danger.

The mobility component   Although the mobility component is given to people who are unable or virtually unable to walk, or need help getting around, you can spend it how you choose. It is not available to people who become disabled, or make a claim, after the age of 65. Local authorities cannot take into account your mobility component when assessing whether, and how much, you need to pay for any care services.

You may receive the higher level if you are unable to walk or have great difficulty in walking without severe discomfort or seriously affecting your health because of a physical disability. The higher level is also available to people who are both registered severely sight-impaired (blind) and assessed as 80% disabled through deafness and need someone with them when they go outdoors; or have lost both legs at or above the ankle (or were born without legs or feet); or are severely mentally impaired and have severe behavioural problems and get the highest rate of the care component.

If you can physically walk but need someone with you most of the time for guidance or supervision when out of doors in unfamiliar places, you may be awarded the lower rate mobility component.

Using a car

If you get the higher rate of the mobility component of DLA, you can apply for road tax exemption for one car. It does not matter whether you are the owner of the car, but the car will have to be used primarily for your benefit to get the exemption. You will get details about this and about using your higher-rate mobility component to get a car on contract hire or hire purchase through the Motability scheme when you first get the allowance (see page 208 for Motability's address).

You can also apply to your local authority for a Blue Badge (previously an Orange Badge), which allows parking with some limitations but without charge at meters or where waiting is restricted. This can be used in any car in which you are travelling. Some local authorities make a small charge for issuing the badge.

Examples of people who may receive DLA or AA

Ellen is 62 and cannot walk very far owing to severe osteo-arthritis in her hips and hands. Although she can manage to care for herself, she finds cooking very difficult because she cannot do tasks such as cutting, lifting and pouring. She applied for DLA and was awarded the higher level of the mobility component and the lowest rate of the care component.

Albert is 64 and suffers from dementia. During the day, his wife or another relative stays with him all the time because he is very forgetful and sometimes wanders off or turns on the gas without lighting it. He normally sleeps all through the night. His wife applied for DLA on his behalf and he was awarded the middle rate of the care component (because he needs supervision during the day) and the lower rate of the mobility component because he needs guidance and supervision when outdoors.

Sarah is 68 and had a severe stroke six months ago that left her unable to walk and needing a lot of help – for example, with washing, dressing and eating. Because she is over 65, the rules prevent her from applying for DLA. She cannot get any help with her mobility needs but she can apply for AA because she needs personal care.

Remember that these are just examples and your situation is probably different. Whether you qualify for DLA or AA, and if so at what rate, will depend on your particular circumstances.

Rules covering both AA and DLA

If you are away from home   If you are receiving National Health Service (NHS) treatment in a hospital, you cannot start to receive AA or DLA (although you can make a claim and, if you fulfil the conditions, the allowance can be paid when you go home). However, you may receive either of these allowances if you are a private patient paying for the cost of hospital services.

If you are already receiving AA or DLA and you go into hospital, you will be able to continue to receive the allowance for up to four weeks. However, the allowance will stop sooner if your admission is within 28 days of a previous stay in hospital. The days you are admitted and discharged do not count as days in hospital.

Should you have a current contract with Motability, there are special rules that can enable you to continue to receive payment of the mobility component while in hospital.

Before July 1996, a stay in hospital did not normally affect the mobility component of DLA. Some people in hospital for 12 months or more in July 1996 received transitional protection and can continue to get an amount equivalent to the lower rate of the mobility component.

FOR MORE INFORMATION about AA and DLA for people in care homes, see pages 144–147.

Living abroad   In general you need to be ordinarily resident in the UK and present here when you make your claim, and (unless you are applying under the special rules for terminally ill people) have been here or in the Isle of Man, Jersey or Guernsey for at least 26 weeks of the last 12 months.

In general, temporary absence abroad for up to six months does not affect AA or DLA, nor do periods abroad taken specifically for medical treatment. You should let your pension centre know when you intend to go abroad.

You may be able to keep AA or DLA if you go to live permanently in another EEA country. You usually need also to be entitled to a state pension or certain other benefits from the UK (including industrial injuries benefit, incapacity benefit, contribution-based ESA or a bereavement benefit) to be able to export your AA or DLA.

FOR THE LATEST INFORMATION about people who currently live in the European Economic Area (EEA) or Switzerland, or who move there, go to the Direct Gov website (at www.direct.gov.uk/en/DisabledPeople/ FinancialSupport/Introductiontofinancialsupport/ DG_073387).

The exportability team at PDCS deals with claims for disability benefits from people who live in, or are moving to, another country in the EEA or Switzerland. Their address is: Exportability Co-ordinator, Room C216, Pension, Disability and Carers Service, Warbreck House, Blackpool, FY2 0YE.

How to claim

You can get the claim form for AA (AA1) or DLA (DLA1):

- by telephoning the Benefit Enquiry Line on 0800 88 22 00 (textphone: 0800 24 33 55);
- by sending off the tear-off slip from the leaflets AA or DLA;
- from some local advice agencies; or
- on the Direct Gov website (www.direct.gov.uk/disability).You can also claim online from this website.

If the forms are sent to you because you contacted the Benefit Enquiry Line, from a DWP office or because you returned the tear-off slip, they will be dated. As long as you return the form in the envelope provided within six weeks, your claim, if successful, will start on the day your request was received. If you get the claim pack from a local advice agency, unless it has been designated as an 'Alternative Office', this will not normally be dated and the claim will start from the date the completed form is received by the Disability and Carers Service.

The intention is that you can describe how your disability affects you on the form and that a medical examination will not normally be necessary. Although changes have been made to improve the forms, they are still quite long and you may want some assistance with filling them in.

You can get help to fill in the form from a friend or relative or a local advice agency, or you can phone the Benefits Enquiry Line on 0800 88 22 00 (free call). If it is difficult for you to get out, you can ask for someone to visit to help you with the form.

If you have difficulty completing the claim form and would rather have a medical examination, you can ask for a doctor to visit.

FOR MORE INFORMATION, contact The Disability Alliance (address on page 206), which produces guides to help people claim AA and DLA.

When filling in the form, remember that it does not matter if you actually receive any help or not. Be sure to say what activities are difficult or impossible for you. For example, you may have to get dressed on your own because there is no one to help you, but do explain if it takes a long time or if it is difficult. If you feel that having answered the questions you have not given a good picture of how your disability affects you, add any extra information you think would be helpful. If you have any problems with filling in the form, do ask for help. There is also a space on the form for your doctor or someone else who knows about your circumstances to complete.

If your claim cannot be decided from the information in

the form, someone from the Disability and Carers Service may phone you for more information, ask for further information from someone such as your doctor or community nurse, or arrange a medical examination.

If an appointment is made for a doctor to visit, you may want a friend or relative to be present at that time. This will be particularly important if you have difficulty making yourself understood. The doctor, who will not be your own doctor but one appointed by the DWP, will probably examine you and ask further questions. It may be useful to make a note beforehand of the things you need to tell the doctor about when you need help or the difficulties you experience.

When to claim   Although you normally need to fulfil the qualifying conditions for three months before you can start getting DLA and six months for AA, if you have only recently become disabled, you should still apply straight away, as it may take some weeks to deal with your claim.

If you are receiving a lower level of one of the allowances, but your condition has deteriorated so you might now qualify for a higher level, you can ask for your case to be reconsidered. You will need to satisfy the care or mobility conditions for the higher level for three months (DLA) or six months (AA) before it can be paid.

You should be aware that, if you ask for your case to be looked at again, there is a possibility that instead of awarding a higher level your benefit might be stopped or reduced. You may want to seek help from a local advice agency to discuss your position and to ensure that you include all the relevant information if you ask for your benefit to be reconsidered.

Terminal illness   People who are terminally ill can claim DLA or AA without the three-month or six-month waiting period, under 'Special Rules' that make the application process quicker and simpler. You will be considered to be terminally ill if you have a progressive illness that is likely to limit your life expectancy to six months or less.

To claim, ask your doctor for a DS1500 report, which gives details of your condition. If you are sending the DS1500 report with the AA or DLA form, make sure that you have ticked the Special Rules box. You will not need to complete the whole form – information next to the special rules box explains which parts you need to fill in. Then sign the claim form and send it, and the DS1500, in the envelope provided.

If you are awarded benefit under the Special Rules, you will automatically receive the higher rate of AA or the highest level of the care component of DLA. However, if you are under the age of 65 and you want to claim the mobility component of DLA, you will need to fill in the mobility-related sections as part of your claim. Claims should be handled within 10 to 14 days and a medical examination will not normally be necessary.

An application can be made by another person, on behalf of someone who is terminally ill, with or without their knowledge, so it is possible for people to receive an allowance under the Special Rules without knowing their prognosis.

Effect on other benefits Entitlement to AA or DLA can also enable you to get a higher amount of other benefits such as Pension Credit, Income Support, income-based Jobseeker's Allowance (JSA), income-related ESA, Housing Benefit or Council Tax Benefit. You will need to make a separate claim for these benefits and you may be able to receive payments backdated to the time your disability benefit started. If you are not sure of your position, get help from a local advice agency.

How it is paid AA or DLA may be awarded indefinitely or for a set period, in which case it will be reviewed at the end of this time. If your allowance is awarded for a fixed period, you should be sent a renewal claim about six months before the end of the award. There is a 'Right Payment Programme' for DLA recipients, which means that you may be sent a questionnaire or receive a visit to check if your needs are still the same.

AA is normally paid four-weekly in arrears directly into a bank, building society or other account. If payment into an account is not suitable for you, weekly cheques will be sent in the post (see pages 19–20 for more information). If you are receiving another benefit or pension, they will normally be paid together. DLA is normally paid four-weekly in arrears. However, people claiming either AA or DLA under the Special Rules because they are terminally ill can get weekly payments in advance.

If you disagree with a decision If you disagree with a decision about your allowance, you can ask for the decision to be reconsidered or make an appeal. You will be sent details about how to do this when you receive the decision. It is important to challenge a decision or get advice as quickly as possible because there are time limits that generally mean you must take action within one month – see pages 42–43 for more information or look at the *Disability Rights Handbook*, which has more detailed information (see page 211).

> FOR MORE INFORMATION, *see Age UK factsheets* Attendance Allowance *and* Disability Living Allowance; *for AA, see DWP leaflet* Attendance Allowance *and claim form AA1; for DLA, see DWP leaflet* Disability Living Allowance *and claim form DLA1.*

CARER'S ALLOWANCE

Carer's Allowance (which used to be called Invalid Care Allowance) is a benefit for people who are caring for a severely disabled person for at least 35 hours a week.

The benefit does not depend on having paid NI contributions. Carer's Allowance is taxable.

Do note that in some situations the person you care for could lose money if you start to receive Carer's Allowance. This could happen if the person you care for receives the severe disability premium or extra amount for severe disability as part of their Pension Credit, Income Support, income-related ESA, Housing Benefit or Council Tax Benefit. (See pages 55–57 for more information about the severe disability premium/addition.)

The weekly rates are:

Carer	£53.90
Adult dependant	£31.70

From 6 April 2010, no new adult dependant increases will be awarded, and from April 2020 they will be abolished altogether. If you were entitled to an adult dependant increase before 2010, you will continue to receive it until 2020 (unless entitlement stops for some other reason).

The person being cared for must be receiving one of the benefits referred to below. They do not have to be a relative and may live separately or with you. Entitlement to Carer's Allowance may continue for up to eight weeks after the death of the person being cared for.

Who qualifies?

To qualify you must spend at least 35 hours a week looking after someone who is receiving AA (higher or lower rate), the care component of DLA (middle or highest rate), or CAA of £58.40 or more paid with an industrial injuries disablement, war or service pension.

There is no upper age limit for claiming Carer's Allowance, although if you are receiving a State Pension or another benefit, you may not receive any or all of the allowance on top of this.

Carer's Allowance can be backdated for up to three months (provided the qualifying conditions have been met throughout that time).

It can be backdated for a longer period if the disabled person who receives the care has only recently been awarded AA, middle or highest rate DLA care component, or CAA. As long as you claim Carer's Allowance within three months of the disabled person being awarded a qualifying benefit, your entitlement to Carer's Allowance will start from the same date as the disabled person's entitlement to that qualifying benefit.

You cannot get Carer's Allowance if you earn more than £100 a week after the deduction of allowable expenses such as income tax and NI contributions. The extra £31.70 that can be claimed for a dependent adult will not be paid if that person earns more than £31.70 a week, including any occupational or personal pension. It also may not be paid if they are receiving a State Pension or certain other benefits. When calculating the net earnings of the carer or their partner, certain work expenses are deducted.

Protecting your State Pension

If you are entitled to Carer's Allowance, NI contributions will be credited automatically to protect your right to a future State Pension, unless you have retained the right to pay the married woman's reduced-rate contributions. Entitlement to Carer's Allowance can also help you build up State Second Pension, as explained on page 23, and if you become sick, you may qualify for ESA based on NI credits from when you were receiving Carer's Allowance.

If you are a carer, but do not qualify for Carer's Allowance (perhaps because the person you look after does not get DLA or AA, or you do not care for them for 35 hours a week), you may still be able to qualify for carer's NI credit. Carer's NI credits are available to people getting Child

Benefit for a child under 12, registered foster carers and people spending 20 hours a week or more caring for a severely disabled person.

FOR MORE INFORMATION go to the Direct Gov website (at http://www.direct.gov.uk/en/CaringForSomeone/ MoneyMatters/DG_10038111).

Overlap with the State Pension and increases to other benefits

If you are already getting £53.90 a week or more from other social security benefits or State Pensions, you may not be able to get Carer's Allowance as well. This is because it 'overlaps' with some benefits, including Incapacity Benefit, Contributory ESA, State Pension and Widow's Pension. If you have a spouse, civil partner or partner who is claiming an addition to their benefit for you, that addition will be reduced by the amount of Carer's Allowance you receive.

However, if you have a low income, it may still be worth claiming Carer's Allowance even though it may not be paid. Although Carer's Allowance is counted as income if you claim Pension Credit, Income Support, income-related ESA, Housing Benefit or Council Tax Benefit, people entitled to Carer's Allowance may be able to get higher rates of these benefits because of the 'carer premium' (extra amount for caring in Pension Credit).

Example

Olive is 62 and looks after her mother who gets AA. Olive has no savings and has a total income of £137.65 (State Pension of £97.65 and an occupational pension of £40 a week). She is not entitled to Pension Credit because her income is more than £132.60 – the basic Pension Credit level for someone of her age.

She applies for Carer's Allowance but, although she satisfies the conditions, it cannot be paid because her

State Pension is more than £53.90 – the level of Carer's Allowance. However, because she is entitled to Carer's Allowance (even though it is not paid) her Pension Credit rate is now £162.65 – the basic rate of £132.60 plus the carer addition of £30.05. She is now entitled to £25.00 in Pension Credit to bring her pensions of £137.65 up to the Pension Credit rate.

Carer's Allowance after State Pension age

If you are receiving Carer's Allowance when you reach State Pension age (see page 35), it will be adjusted to take account of your Pension. If your State Pension is £53.90 or more, payment of Carer's Allowance will stop. If your State Pension is less than £53.90, Carer's Allowance will be reduced by the amount of State Pension you receive. If you are not entitled to a State Pension or do not claim one, Carer's Allowance may continue to be paid in full.

If you were 65 or over on 28 October 2002 and receiving Invalid Care Allowance when the upper age limit for claiming was abolished, you may be able to continue to receive Carer's Allowance even if you are no longer caring. Otherwise, the allowance will stop when you are no longer caring or up to eight weeks later if the person you care for dies.

How to claim

To make a claim you will need claim pack DS700 or DS700(SP) if you receive a State Pension. You can get these packs from your local Jobcentre Plus office, by ringing the Benefit Enquiry Line on 0800 88 22 00 (free call) or the Carer's Allowance claim pack order line on 01772 899729 (textphone: 01772 562202), or from the Direct Gov website (www.direct.gov.uk) where you can also claim online. In Northern Ireland, phone 028 90 906186; you cannot claim online.

FOR MORE INFORMATION, see Age UK factsheet Carer's Allowance *and DWP leaflet CAA5DCS* Carer's

Allowance. *Carers UK produces information for carers – see page 206 for the address.*

STATUTORY SICK PAY

Statutory Sick Pay (SSP) is paid by employers to employees who satisfy the qualifying conditions for payment. If you are unable to work because of sickness but you are self-employed or unemployed, you may be entitled to ESA, as explained below.

If you are an employee and you have been off sick for at least four days in a row (including weekends and bank holidays) and you have earnings of at least £97 a week, you may be entitled to SSP. Your earnings are averaged over an eight-week period before your sickness began. This period may be different if you are paid weekly or monthly or at other times. SSP is not payable for the first three days of sickness and is usually paid for the days that you would normally work.

There is no upper age limit. SSP can continue for up to 28 weeks and will be paid by your employer. SSP is taxable. The weekly rate is £79.15. You may also get sick pay from your employer's own scheme, depending on their terms and conditions.

If your SSP has come to an end or you are not entitled to SSP, your employer must give you form SSP1 to help support your claim to ESA, as explained below. If you are under the Pension Credit qualifying age (see below) and receiving SSP, you may also be entitled to some Income Support if your SSP is not enough to live on. If you are over the Pension Credit qualifying age and receiving SSP, you may be able to claim Pension Credit.

EMPLOYMENT AND SUPPORT ALLOWANCE

This is a benefit for people who are unable to work because of illness or disability. Introduced on 27 October 2008, it replaced Incapacity Benefit and Income Support on the basis of incapacity for new applicants from that date onwards. ESA has both a means-tested and an NI-based element.

Contributory ESA is paid if you have enough recent NI contributions. It is not generally means-tested, but if you receive a personal or occupational pension of more than £85 a week, your ESA may be reduced, as explained below.

Income-related ESA is for people who do not have enough contributions to receive contributory ESA, or for people receiving contributory ESA but whose ESA is not enough to live on.

> FOR MORE INFORMATION, see the Disability Alliance Guide to Employment and Support Allowance (see page 206). There is also information on the Direct Gov website (www.direct.gov.uk).

ESA is available only to people making a new claim from 27 October 2008. If you were already receiving Incapacity Benefit, Severe Disablement Allowance (SDA) or Income Support on the basis of incapacity before then, you will continue to receive those benefits. The Government intends to 'migrate' people on those benefits onto ESA over the next few years. Some people who have been on Incapacity Benefit since 1995 have transitional protection and some of the rules apply to them differently. See page 123 about the rules for people who were transferred from Invalidity Benefit to Incapacity Benefit in April 1995.

ESA has been introduced because the Government wants to make sure that sick or disabled people are encouraged to consider what steps they could take to get back to work. People receiving ESA will be put into one of two groups that will determine how much they have to prepare for work as a condition of receiving benefit. People in the work-related activity group will have a series of meetings with a personal adviser and will be offered support to consider what work they may be able to do in the future. If they do not comply with the recommendations made in these meetings, or take part fully, their benefit could be reduced. The most severely disabled people will be put in the support group. They will not have to engage in work-related activities and will receive a higher rate of benefit.

The weekly rates of ESA for people over 25 are:

Basic personal allowance

Single (contributory and income-related ESA)	£65.45
Couple (income-related ESA only)	£102.75
Work-related activity component (paid after assessment period)	£25.95
Support component (paid after assessment period)	£31.40

When you first claim ESA you will begin a 13-week assessment period. During this time you will have a medical examination, be put either into the support group or the work-related activity group, and you will usually have an initial interview with a personal adviser about the sorts of work you could do.

During the assessment phase you will receive the single rate of the basic personal allowance if you are claiming contributory ESA. If you are claiming income-related ESA, you will receive either the single or the couple rate of ESA personal allowance plus any premiums you might be entitled to.

After the assessment phase you will be put into either the support group or the work-related activity group and you will receive the extra component for that group (note that there is no couple rate of either component).

Income-related ESA premiums

Enhanced disability

Single	£13.65
Couple	£19.65

This is paid either where the ESA claimant is placed in the support group, or if either the claimant or their partner receives the higher rate of DLA care component.

Severe disability

one qualifies	£53.65
couple both qualify	£107.30

This is paid where:

- the claimant is receiving DLA middle or higher rate care component;
- no one is being paid Carer's Allowance for looking after them;
- the claimant lives alone or, if the claimant has a partner, they both receive DLA middle or higher rate care component, or their partner is registered blind (for more information about this premium, see 'Pension Credit', pages 55–56).

Carer

For each person who qualifies	£30.05

This is paid when the claimant or their partner is entitled to Carer's Allowance.

Contributory Employment and Support Allowance

To qualify for ESA you must have a limited capability for work and be under State Pension age (see page 35) when your period of incapacity began.

You must normally also have paid enough NI contributions in one of the last three tax years. If you have recently been receiving Carer's Allowance, contributions paid more than three years ago may enable you to qualify. Some young people may qualify for ESA without needing to satisfy the contribution conditions if their disability began before the age of 25.

Income-related Employment and Support Allowance

This may be paid if you are under State Pension age, have a limited capability for work and either you do not have enough NI contributions to get contributory ESA or your contributory ESA is not enough to live on.

The medical tests for Employment and Support Allowance

When you initially claim ESA you will need to supply a medical certificate from a doctor. During the 13-week assessment phase the DWP will assess your capacity for work. There are three medical tests for ESA:

1 **Limited capability for work**   This is the test that determines whether you will be entitled to ESA. It assesses your ability to carry out specific everyday activities. This relates to physical, mental and sensory functions, and includes activities such as walking, lifting and carrying, hearing, seeing, interacting with other people and coping with changes in your daily routine. There is a points system to assess problems with these aspects. You have to score at least 15 points to be assessed as having a limited capacity for work. You will normally complete an ESA 50 form listing the problems you have, and you will then be examined by a health practitioner working for the DWP at a medical examination centre.

2 **Limited capability for work-related activity**   This test decides whether you will go into the work-related activity group or the support group. The Government expects that most claimants will be put into the work-related activity group.

3 **Work-focused health-related assessment**   This assessment is only done for people in the work-related activity group. It looks at the sort of activities

you can do and what help you might need to get back into work. It will be used by your personal adviser to plan what activities you might have to do while you are on ESA.

Work and ESA Normally if you do any work you will not be entitled to ESA, Incapacity Benefit or Severe Disablement Allowance (SDA). However, there are certain sorts of 'permitted work' you can do and remain entitled to ESA, Incapacity Benefit or SDA. Under the Permitted Work rules you can work for up to 16 hours a week and earn up to £93.00 a week, but you can only do this for up to 52 weeks.

If you continue to work after 52 weeks, you will only be allowed to earn up to £20. If you earn more than this, the work will not be accepted as 'permitted work'. This 52-week time limit does not apply if you are in the support group of ESA, or if you are doing 'supported permitted work'. Supported permitted work means work that is supervised by someone who is employed by a public or local authority or a voluntary organisation, and whose job it is to arrange work for disabled people. This could be work done in the community or in a sheltered workshop. It also includes work as part of a hospital treatment programme.

The figure of £93.00 is based on 16 hours' work at the minimum wage, and may increase in October 2010 if the minimum wage rises.

You must tell the DWP that you are working. For more information, contact your Jobcentre Plus office.

Occupational and personal pensions Your contributory ESA and Incapacity Benefit may be reduced if you have an occupational, stakeholder or personal pension of more than £85 a week. For every £1 of pension more than £85, you will lose 50p of benefit. Your Incapacity Benefit will not be reduced if you have been receiving it since before 6 April

2001 or if you receive the highest rate of the care component of DLA.

When you reach State Pension age you will no longer be entitled to ESA and should claim your State Pension.

People still receiving Incapacity Benefit People who were already receiving Incapacity Benefit, SDA or Income Support on the basis of incapacity before 27 October 2008 will remain on those benefits, but the Government does intend that they will be moved onto ESA, and the new medical tests applied to them, at some point in the future.

Incapacity Benefit rates for 2010 are:

Short-term lower rate (under State Pension age)	£68.95
Short-term higher rate (under State Pension age)	£81.60
Long-term rate	£91.40

If you became unable to work before the age of 45, you receive an age addition paid with long-term Incapacity Benefit. There are two rates, depending on the age at which you become unable to work:

Under 35	£15.00
35–44	£5.80

The Government intends to align the rates of Incapacity Benefit and ESA. To achieve this, the Incapacity Benefit age additions from 2010 have been reduced, so that people receiving the long-term rate with an age addition will see their total Incapacity Benefit increase by less than the rate of increase in other benefits.

Increases in Incapacity Benefit for a husband, wife or civil partner Your Incapacity Benefit may include an increase for your husband, wife or civil partner, or for a person who looks after your children. You may be entitled to an increase for an adult dependant if your husband, wife or civil partner is over State Pension age. If you are receiving the long-term rate of Incapacity Benefit, the increase for a dependant is £53.10 a week. If you are receiving either of the short-term rates, and you are under State Pension age, the increase is £41.35.

However, these increases 'overlap' with any State Pension or certain other State benefits that your dependant is receiving. So if, for example, you are a married man and your wife has a State Pension of £60 a week, you would not be entitled to an increase for her. If her State Pension were £25 a week, the amount you could receive would be reduced by £25.

If your spouse or civil partner has earnings of more than £65.45 a week (if you are getting the long-term rate) or £41.35 a week (for the short-term rate), you cannot receive an adult dependency increase – any occupational or personal pension your spouse/civil partner receives will be counted as earnings.

The long-term rate of Incapacity Benefit cannot be paid after State Pension age. So once you reach State Pension age (see page 35), you should claim the State Pension. It will be worked out as explained in the section starting on page 2, although if you were receiving an age addition with your Incapacity Benefit, this can be paid with your State Pension as an invalidity addition (after the deduction of any additional State Pension and contracted-out deductions).

For people over State Pension age the short-term lower rate of Incapacity Benefit is £87.75 a week and the higher rate is £91.40, although you may get less if you do not have enough contributions for a full basic State Pension. You may also receive additional State Pension and Graduated Retirement Benefit. There is an adult dependency increase of £51.10, which you may receive if your husband, wife or civil partner is State Pension age or over – depending on any earnings, pensions or other benefits they receive.

From 6 April 2010 no new adult dependant increases will be awarded, and they will be abolished altogether from April 2020. If you were entitled to an adult dependant increase before April 2010, you will continue to receive it until 2020 (unless entitlement stops for some other reason).

If you were receiving Invalidity Benefit on 12 April 1995

You may receive an extra Invalidity Allowance if you were previously getting it with your Invalidity Benefit. The rates, which depend on the age at which you became unable to work, are:

Under 40	£15.00
40–49	£8.40
Men 50–59, women 50–54	£5.45

Some people also receive an Additional Rate based on any entitlement to additional State Pension built up between 1978 and 1991. This is paid at a frozen amount and 'overlaps' with Invalidity Allowance. In other respects the Incapacity Benefit rules are generally the same as those described on page 121.

How to claim

To claim ESA, contact your local Jobcentre Plus office. People claiming ESA (and other benefits for people of working age) will normally be required to attend some work-focused interviews as a condition of benefit. The aim is to look at work options, as well as to provide information about what practical and financial help is available.

If you disagree with a decision

If you disagree with a decision about your benefit, you can ask for the decision to be revised or you can make an appeal, as explained on pages 42–43.

SEVERE DISABLEMENT ALLOWANCE

SDA was abolished for new claimants on 6 April 2001. However, you can still receive it if you were entitled to the benefit on or before 5 April 2001 and have been receiving it continuously since then (although short breaks may be covered by certain linking rules). If you are already in receipt of SDA, it can still be paid as long as you continue to satisfy the entitlement conditions. It was a benefit for people who were incapable of working but who did not have enough contributions to get Incapacity Benefit.

SDA is not based on NI contributions and is not taxable. The basic weekly rates are:

Claimant	£59.45
Adult dependant	£31.90

There are also additions for people who became unable to work before State Pension age; these are added to the basic rate of £59.45. The weekly rates are:

Under 40	£15.00
40–49	£8.40
50-59	£5.45

SDA is not means-tested but is taken into account if you apply for income-related benefits such as Income Support or Pension Credit. Contact a local advice agency or write to Age UK at the address on page 224 if you need more information about SDA.

Since 13 April 1995 the adult dependency increase for your husband or wife (or civil partner) has been payable only if they are State Pension age or over. The amount is £31.90 per week. If they have earnings over £65.45 or receive a State Pension or other benefit of £31.90 or more, you may not be able to get this increase. If you have been receiving the increase since before 13 April 1995, it can continue, even if your husband, wife or civil partner is under State Pension age.

From 6 April 2010, no new adult dependant increases will be awarded, and they will be abolished altogether from April 2020. If you were entitled to an adult dependant increase before April 2010, you will continue to receive it until 2020 (unless entitlement stops for some other reason).

SDA can continue to be paid after you reach State Pension age, but the 'overlapping benefit' rules apply, which means that it is not paid in addition to certain other State Pensions or benefits. You cannot receive both the full amount of SDA and a State Pension. If you do not qualify for a State Pension or it is less than SDA, you can continue to receive SDA.

OTHER BENEFITS FOR PEOPLE WITH DISABILITIES

This section gives brief information about other benefits for people with disabilities. More detailed information is given in the leaflets mentioned or you could look at the *Disability Rights Handbook* (see page 211).

Industrial injuries scheme

The industrial injuries scheme can provide help to people who are disabled as a result of an accident at work or an industrial disease.

The main benefit is Disablement Benefit, which can be paid in addition to other NI benefits such as Incapacity Benefit/ESA or State Pension. The level of payment depends on how disabled you are assessed as being.

If you are awarded Disablement Benefit at the 100% rate, you may also qualify for Constant Attendance Allowance (CAA) if you need care and attention. There is also an Exceptionally Severe Disablement Allowance for those who are likely to need high levels of attention on a permanent basis.

FOR MORE INFORMATION, see leaflet DWP1004 Industrial Injuries Disablement Benefits and other compensation schemes.

War pensions

You may be entitled to some financial help if you are disabled (physically or mentally) or widowed as a result of service in the UK Armed Forces. You may get a tax-free lump sum or a pension. Civilians may also be entitled to financial help in some circumstances.

If you need care and attention because of your pensioned disablement, you may also receive CAA and a Mobility Supplement if you have difficulty walking.

FOR MORE INFORMATION about war pensions, ring the Veterans Helpline on 0800 169 2277 (free call). You can also ask for details of your nearest War Pensioner's Welfare Service. This is an advice and support service for all war pensioners and war widows/widowers/ surviving civil partners living in the UK. The Welfare Service also gives advice and assistance to anyone who has served in the UK Armed Forces.

Ex-gratia payments for British groups held prisoner by the Japanese in the Second World War Some British people and in some cases their widows or widowers are entitled to a single ex-gratia payment of £10,000. These payments are not taken into account for income-related benefits.

FOR MORE INFORMATION, contact the Veterans Helpline on 0800 169 2277 (free call).

PAYING FOR CARE

This section explains the help you can get with paying for the costs of care in all settings. This might be care at home (such as personal care or domestic help in your home, day

126

care or a night sitting service) or care in a care home. It covers people living in England, Scotland and Wales. Although the system in Northern Ireland is broadly similar, there are a number of differences, so contact Age Northern Ireland at the address on page 224 if you need more information.

Many people buy their own care without social services' help. This section looks at the help you can receive from social services and how you may be charged for that help. There are national rules for charging for care in care homes, but each local authority is able to decide whether and how much to charge for care to help you remain at home, subject to certain minimum requirements.

Applying for help with care

If you need help with your care, either to help you to remain at home or if you think you might need to move into a care home, you can ask for an assessment of your needs by the local authority (the county, metropolitan or London borough or unitary authority). The adult social services department (social work department in Scotland) will be responsible for arranging an assessment of your care needs.

After this assessment the local authority will decide whether you are entitled to any help either to enable you to remain in your own home, to explore other housing options or to move into a care home. Each local authority has its own criteria for making these decisions within a national framework. Some local authorities have a ceiling on the amount of care (either the number of hours or the cost) they will provide to help you remain at home. If you do not agree with the decision, you can make a complaint through the complaints procedure.

It may be beneficial for you to request an assessment even if you will eventually have to fund any services that you receive. Your right to an assessment does not relate to your resources because the local authority's duty to assess is triggered by your needs and potential eligibility for service provision.

In England and Wales your carer (if you have one) is entitled to an assessment in their own right and to services that will help them care for you. They have a right to an assessment of their needs even if you do not want to be assessed. In Scotland a carer is entitled to an assessment of their needs, which will be taken into account in deciding the services the person being cared for is offered.

> *FOR MORE INFORMATION about local authority assessment for community care services in England and Wales, contact Age UK Advice on 0800 169 65 65. In Scotland, call the Scottish Helpline for Older People (SHOP) on 0845 125 9732. In Northern Ireland, call Age NI Advice on 0808 808 7575.*

PAYING FOR CARE AT HOME

This section looks at the help you can receive either from local authorities through direct payments or from the Independent Living Fund in paying for care to help you remain at home. It then explains the rules that a local authority uses when working out how much to charge you for care it has provided or arranged for you.

Direct payments

Local authorities can give people cash payments as an alternative to arranging community care services for them. Local authorities have to offer direct payments to older people who meet the eligibility requirements. You can choose this option if it best suits your needs.

You can choose to employ a carer yourself, or use a local home care agency if you do not wish to take on the responsibility of being an employer. You may find that there is a support group in your area to help people with managing direct payments. Carers in England and Wales are also able to receive direct payments instead of the services that can be provided for them.

To get a direct payment you generally have to be able to manage the payments, alone or with assistance. In Scotland people who manage your affairs, such as an attorney or guardian, can have a direct payment (which is also known as self-directed support in Scotland). In England and Wales direct payments cannot usually be used to pay a spouse or close relative in the same household unless the local authority thinks this is the most appropriate way of meeting your needs. In Scotland, updated guidance has been introduced that allows close relatives to be employed if the local authority is satisfied that this is necessary and appropriate. The local authority has to monitor that the money is being spent on the care you need. If you want a direct payment but your local authority refuses, you can use the complaints procedure.

In November 2009, new Government Regulations extended eligibility for direct payments to certain adults who lack capacity and to those who are subject to certain restrictions under mental health legislation. Direct payments can now be made to a willing and appropriate 'suitable person', such as a family member or friend, who receives and manages the payments on behalf of the person who lacks capacity. Government guidance to local authorities describes the process to be followed for appointing a suitable person, and the conditions and standards that they must meet to fulfil this role. It also provides advice on dispute resolution.

FOR MORE INFORMATION about direct payments in England and Wales, contact your local authority or

Age UK Advice on 0800 169 65 65. In Scotland, call the Scottish Personal Assistant Employers Network (SPAEN) on 01698 250280 or the Scottish Helpline for Older People (SHOP) on 0845 125 9732. In Northern Ireland, call Age NI Advice on 0808 808 7575.

Personal budgets and individual budgets

The Government is developing personal budgets as part of its 'personalisation' agenda in social care. A personal budget is a sum of money allocated to an individual who is assessed as needing personal assistance services. They were first introduced in April 2008 as part of the Government's programme of transforming social care. These payments have still to be introduced in Northern Ireland.

Personal budgets are a form of self-directed support similar to direct payments, which are intended to increase service users' choice and control over the services they receive. They are an upfront allocation of social care funding that individuals can use innovatively.

You can take this funding in the form of direct payments or you can continue to have the local authority pay directly for the care you need, or a combination of both. It can be a cash payment, or it can be a 'virtual' budget that is managed for you, but you know upfront how much money there is to spend over a year and decide with a support worker (also known as a broker) how you wish to design your care package to meet your identified needs.

The key features of a personal budget are:

- a transparent allocation of resources so that you know how much you have to spend on your support;
- the opportunity to use the budget in ways that best suit you;

- you can have the support of brokers, advocates or user-led organisations to help you develop your support plan and manage it;
- the funding can be paid to you in a number of ways, depending on the amount of support you need to arrange your care.

At present personal budgets are not intended to be used for long-term residential care, but this may be included in the future.

The Government has also piloted the use of individual budgets, which are similar to personal budgets in their aim of increasing service users' choice and control over the services they receive. However, they are intended to allow access to a number of local authority funding streams beyond those for personal assistance services to create a single individual budget. Examples may include the use of funding streams for Access to Work, Community Equipment and Housing Support.

The main focus of Government policy in England at the moment relates to the introduction of personal budgets rather than individual budgets. Research findings from the Association of Directors of Adult Social Services shows that by March 2009, 93,000 people were receiving personal budgets (40% of whom were older people), and it is hoped that by March 2010 this figure will reach 206,000.

The focus of Government policy in Scotland aims to encourage a flexible approach to personal budgets, making it easier for them to fit local circumstances and need, and supporting co-operative working from a range of agencies outside social work departments.

FOR MORE INFORMATION about personal and individual budgets in England see the Age UK factsheet Self-directed Support: Direct Payments, Personal Budgets and Individual Budgets. *Or go to*

*the In-Control website (www.in-control.org.uk), the
Department of Health website (www.dh.gov.uk/en/
SocialCare/Socialcarereform/personalisation/individual
budgets/index.htm) or the National Centre for
Independent Living website (www.ncil.org.uk).
For information in Scotland, go to Self-Directed
Scotland's website (www.sdsscotland.org.uk)*

The Independent Living Fund

The Independent Living Fund (2006) (ILF) provides
discretionary cash payments to enable disabled people
with high support needs to pay for personal care or help
with household tasks in order to remain living at home.

You can be considered for help from the ILF if you are
under 65 years of age when your application is received
and have less than £23,000 in savings. You must be
receiving the highest rate care component of DLA, and be
receiving services or cash from the local authority,
currently to the value of at least £320.00 a week. Priority is
given if you are in paid work or self-employed for at least
16 hours a week. Priority is then given if (a) you receive
Income Support, income-related ESA, income-based
Jobseeker's Allowance or Pension Credit Guarantee Credit,
or you are not able to afford the care you need from your
income; and (b) your requirements for care amount to at
least £500.00 a week (jointly funded by the ILF and the
local authority). The maximum weekly payment from the
ILF is £475.00.

*FOR MORE INFORMATION about the Independent
Living Fund call the ILF on 0845 601 8815 or go to the
ILF website (www.ilf.org.uk).*

Charges for care at home

Each local authority has discretion about whether it will
charge people who receive care either provided or

arranged by the local authority. Direct payments and personal budgets are charged for in the same way as other non-residential services. Very few authorities do not charge anything.

In Scotland personal care is free if you are 65 or over, but you may still be charged for non-personal care services.

In Northern Ireland charging procedures for the Home Help service are set out in Circular HSS (SS)1/80. This service is provided free of charge to those over the age of 75.

Any services arranged under Section 117 of the Mental Health Act 1983 for aftercare following detention in hospital must be free (though in Scotland the different laws mean that these services may be chargeable if they are not within the definition of personal care).

Any services arranged by the NHS, such as visits by a community nurse, are also free. If you need NHS continuing healthcare in your own home, both the health element and the social care element come under the NHS and so are free (see below).

In England and Wales if your care comes under the definition of Intermediate Care (in other words, to avoid your having to go into hospital or when you have just come out of hospital), it will be free for six weeks and in certain circumstances this can be extended.

In Scotland you get free services for four weeks when you come out of hospital (even if some of the care is non-personal care). After four weeks, support from the local authority is means-tested and you may have to pay something towards the cost of services that are provided.

Any charge you do pay must be 'reasonable' for you to pay, and you have the right to ask the local authority to reduce the amount or waive it altogether. It is important that the local authority is aware if you have extra costs because of your disability – for example extra washing of clothes, having to pay for a gardener or someone to clean the house, or taxis because you cannot use public transport – so that it can take account of these costs. Any charge should be based only on your resources. If you disagree with your charge, you can ask for it to be reviewed or use the local authority's complaints procedure.

The Department of Health issued guidance for England (called *Fairer charging policies for home care and other non-residential social services*) in 2002. This set out a framework that a local authority must use when deciding its charging policies. The Welsh Assembly has also produced guidance under the same name, which it revised in March 2007. The guidance guarantees that individuals are left with at least basic levels of income after they have been charged for the services. In England new guidance relating to personal budgets has been introduced to supplement the 2002 'Fairer Charging' guidance. Local authorities providing personal budgets should have implemented this charging guidance by March 2010.

You should be left with at least £162.50 per week (for a single person of State Pension age or over – the figures vary according to your age), and you should only be charged the full cost of the service if your capital (excluding your home) is above £23,250 in England and Northern Ireland, £22,700 in Scotland or £22,000 in Wales. Some local authorities have set more generous capital limits and/or have set a maximum charge. Any earnings are not taken into account. The local authority should also offer to check that you are getting all the benefits you are entitled to.

In Scotland the Convention of Scottish Local Authorities (CoSLA) has produced guidance on charging older people for 'non-personal' care services, which is available from their website (www.cosla.gov.uk).

FOR MORE INFORMATION about charges for care at home in England and Wales, contact Age UK Advice on 0800 169 65 65. In Scotland, call the Scottish Helpline for Older People (SHOP) on 0845 125 9732. In Northern Ireland, call Age NI Advice on 0808 808 7575.

Supporting People

In England certain support services related to housing needs – such as community alarms and wardens – can be funded through the 'Supporting People' fund. Supporting People is administered by the local authority and payment is made to the housing provider. Charging policies for these services must be in line with the framework of the Fairer Charging guidance (see above), which is used for non-residential services provided by local authorities.

In Scotland Supporting People ceased to exist in April 2008 as a separate fund for housing support needs. Support provision for housing needs is now known simply as Housing Support, although this funding is no longer ring-fenced by local authorities, to allow more flexible support packages to be developed.

FOR MORE INFORMATION on paying for supported accommodation call Age UK Advice on 0800 169 65 65. For information about the Housing Support provision in Scotland, contact the Scottish Helpline for Older People (SHOP) on 0845 125 9732.

Short breaks and respite care

If the local authority arranges short periods in a care home, it can charge in one of two ways as long as the stay is less than eight weeks. It can choose either to have a 'set' charge, which must be reasonable, or to apply the means test used to calculate the charge for care homes (see below). As your stay counts as 'temporary', your home's value will be ignored. If your care break is in hospital, arranged by the NHS, or is part of Intermediate Care, it will be free. Benefits such as AA may be affected, depending on how frequent your care is and how long it lasts.

Paying for care in a care home

This section summarises the help you can get with care home charges. The term 'care home' covers all homes that are registered homes under the Care Standards Act 2000. This includes independent homes and those owned by the local authority and that provide personal and/or nursing care. In England care homes are regulated by the Care Quality Commission. Before the local authority can offer any financial help, you must have an assessment of your needs, as described on pages 127–128.

New Regulations provide for the re-registration of all regulated adult health and social care service providers with the Care Quality Commission in a staged process throughout 2010. Adult social care services are required to re-register on 1 October. This means that present registration under the Care Standards Act 2000 continues until 30 September 2010.

> *PLEASE NOTE that the information in this section does not apply to people who receive their care free under Section 117 of the* Mental Health Act 1983 *(the rules are different in Scotland and are covered under the* Mental Health (Care and Treatment) (Scotland) Act 2003).

In England and Wales the NHS is responsible for the funding of care provided by a registered nurse in a care home providing nursing. In England the previous three-band system for the amount of NHS-funded nursing care was replaced by a single-band system in October 2007. Residents who were previously on the two rates that were lower than the new single weekly rate were moved up to it on 1 October 2007. Residents who were already on the highest of the three bands were allowed to remain on it. The single weekly rate from April 2010 is £108.70.

If you live in Wales contact Age Cymru at the address on page 224 for details of the rate that applies in your area.

In Scotland local authorities put £71.00 towards the cost of nursing care. However, for people aged 65 and over in Scotland personal care costs are also met (set at £156.00 per week). For the latest information phone the Scottish Helpline for Older People (SHOP) on 0845 125 9732.

In Northern Ireland the weekly amount for people who either self-fund their nursing care or are assessed to pay nursing care fees at the full rate is £100. The issue of free personal care is still being considered.

At the same time that the new registered nursing care rules were implemented, a new framework and decision support tool was introduced for the assessment of fully funded NHS continuing healthcare. This is where, because of the resident's needs, the full cost of care, including accommodation costs, is paid for by the NHS. You may be eligible for fully funded NHS continuing healthcare where your primary need for care is health based.

As well as the main tool there is a fast-track tool and a checklist. The fast-track tool is designed to allow an urgent response where, for example, a person has a rapidly deteriorating condition. The checklist is to be used by health and social care professionals to assist in the initial decision as to whether a person's needs make them appropriate for a full NHS continuing healthcare assessment.

This is a controversial area and previous legal judgements and reports by the Health Service Ombudsman have in the past highlighted the fact that in many areas eligibility criteria for this funding were set too narrowly and assessment procedures were inadequate. It is very important to check that you have been properly assessed for 'fully funded care', if you feel that you may be eligible for it, before the local authority carries out an assessment for means-tested assistance.

FOR MORE INFORMATION about registered nursing care funding and NHS continuing healthcare, contact Age UK Advice on 0800 169 65 65, the Scottish Helpline for Older People (SHOP) on 0845 125 9732, Age NI Advice on 0808 808 7575 or Age Cymru at the address on page 224.

If you need help with your care home costs, you can get help from the local authority and you may also get benefits from the DWP. In some circumstances AA or DLA can be paid, as explained later.

You should be aware that, although there is an assessment process and national charging procedures for care in care homes, sometimes things do not run as smoothly as described here. For example, there may be delays in obtaining an assessment, or the local authority may not agree to take financial responsibility. If you have problems, a local advice agency may be able to help.

Care arranged by the local authority

If the local authority agrees to arrange a place for you in a private or voluntary care home, it will be responsible for paying the full fee to the home and assessing your income and savings to work out how much you must pay towards the fees. If you are in a local authority home, the local authority uses the same rules to work out how much you should pay towards the cost of a place in the home. See below to find out how your other capital such as property is assessed.

You should be able to choose which home you enter, subject to certain conditions.

If the home you choose is more expensive than the local authority thinks you need, the local authority may arrange this, but you will need to make arrangements for the difference in funding to be paid. The local authority or care home provider is not allowed to make up the difference from your Personal Expenses Allowance. You normally have to make arrangements for a friend or relative to pay the difference on your behalf. In some circumstances (such as when you will eventually be selling your property) you are able to pay the top-up yourself.

The local authority must be able to provide suitable accommodation at its 'usual cost'. This is the cost that it has decided is usually required to pay for the type of accommodation you need. If there is no suitable place at the price the local authority would usually pay for someone with your assessed needs, it will be responsible for paying for a more expensive place to meet your needs. The local authority should not request a top-up in these circumstances.

You may need to enter a home costing more than the 'usual cost' because of the particular nature of your needs. Examples might include higher levels of needs or special diets and extra facilities required for cultural or medical reasons. If so, the local authority should meet the extra expense, even if there are places available at the 'usual cost' in other homes that cannot meet those needs. Seek help if you cannot find a home that is suitable at the local authority price and you are being expected to pay a top-up.

Charging procedures

For the local authority assessment, if you have savings of more than an upper capital limit, you will have to pay the full fee until your savings reach that amount. In England and Northern Ireland the upper capital limit is £23,250, in Wales it is £22,000 and in Scotland it is £22,750. In Scotland if you are 65 or over, your full fee is the accommodation and living costs only, as the local authority meets the personal care (£156 per week) and nursing costs (£71) of the home. If you are under 65, it meets just the nursing costs.

If you are already in a care home and are using up your savings, you should apply to the local authority for help a few months before your savings get down to the capital limit. (See pages 141–142 for how your former home is treated.)

For the local authority assessment, savings under a certain amount are fully disregarded but your income may still be taken into account. Savings between the upper and lower capital limits will be counted as though you have an additional £1 a week income from every £250.00 (or part of £250.00). This is called 'tariff income'. In England and Northern Ireland the lower capital limit is £14,250, in Wales it is £22,000 and in Scotland £14,000.

In carrying out the assessment the local authority will take into account your income, including any Pension Credit that you are entitled to. Pension Credit is also assessed on your income and savings but the rules are different in some respects. For Pension Credit the first £10,000 of savings are ignored and every £500.00 (or part of £500.00) over £10,000 will be assumed to produce an income of £1 a week. If you have reached the Pension Credit qualifying age (see page 46), you may be able to claim Pension Credit Guarantee Credit while you are in the care home. You may also qualify for Pension Credit Savings Credit if you are aged 65 or over (see page 63). Your appropriate amount will be calculated in the same way as if you were living in ordinary accommodation.

The local authority calculates how much you should contribute towards the cost of your care by looking at your capital and income (including tariff income). The amount that you are asked to contribute should leave you with a

Personal Expenses Allowance of at least £22.30 a week in England, Northern Ireland and Scotland. In Wales it is £22.50. If you have enough qualifying income to receive Pension Credit Savings Credit, or do not receive this benefit because your qualifying income is too high, you should also be allowed to retain up to £5.75 (£8.60 for couples) per week of that income in addition to the Personal Expenses Allowance.

FOR MORE INFORMATION about local authority charging procedures for care homes, contact Age UK Advice on 0800 169 65 65 in England and Wales. In Scotland, call the Scottish Helpline for Older People (SHOP) on 0845 125 9732. In Northern Ireland, call Age NI Advice on 0808 808 7575.

Owning your home

Local authority assessment   If you are in a care home and you own your own home, its value will normally be taken into account, unless your stay is only temporary, or if your partner, a child under 16 for whom you are responsible, or a 'relative' who is either disabled or State Pension age or over, lives in the property. In addition, the value of your former home (but not of your other capital) is ignored for 12 weeks from the time you become a permanent resident. For the purpose of this disregard, your permanent residence commences from the moment you qualify for financial assistance from the local authority. This is on top of any disregard while your stay was considered temporary. The local authority can also choose to ignore the value of your home if someone else lives there – for example, a friend of State Pension age or over, or a relative or friend under State Pension age who has been caring for you for a substantial period. If the local authority says it will not use this discretion, you might want to complain through the formal complaints procedure.

If the local authority does not ignore the value of your former home (after the initial 12-week disregard), you may be able to enter into a 'deferred payment agreement' with it. In this arrangement the local authority assists you with your fees on a loan basis but places a legal charge on the value of your property so that it can reclaim money owed to it when the property is sold. Government guidance requires local authorities to offer the option of a deferred payment where appropriate. Seek legal advice before entering into a deferred payment agreement.

The local authority is also able to take account of certain assets that you might have transferred to someone else in order to pay less for your care. It may be able to recover any debt from the recipients of such assets if the transfer was made within six months of the local authority arranging the funding of the place in the home. Even if the transfer was made more than six months before, the asset can still be taken into account in the means test for the provision of residential care by the local authority.

FOR MORE INFORMATION about who counts as a relative in this situation and about the treatment of the former home, and to transfer assets and pay for care in a care home in England and Wales, contact Age UK Advice on 0800 169 65 65. In Scotland, call the Scottish Helpline for Older People (SHOP) on 0845 125 9732. In Northern Ireland, call Age NI Advice on 0808 808 7575.

Pension Credit assessment If you move into a care home and are on Pension Credit, let The Pension Service know, as it might make a difference to the amount you receive. If you own your own home, its value will normally be taken into account when your savings are assessed for Pension Credit. However, this value will be ignored for 26 weeks, or longer if reasonable, if you are taking steps to sell it. The value of your home will also be ignored if your spouse or partner lives there, or if a 'relative' who is either disabled or State Pension age or over lives in the property.

The age at which women become eligible for their State Pension is gradually increasing from 60 to 65 between April 2010 and April 2020. This is affecting the qualifying age for both men and women for those social security provisions and concessions that are aligned with women's State Pension age, such as Pension Credit. These changes affect people living in England, Wales and Scotland. Although there is a separate social security system in Northern Ireland, the social security benefits are generally the same. These changes affect Pension Credit and some other social security benefits linked to women's retirement age, and will have an effect on both men and women. It is therefore necessary to be aware of this regarding the means-test arrangements for care home provision. The Government has decided to keep the property-related disregard for relatives living with someone who goes into a care home at 60 years of age.

Couples

When one of a couple enters a care home, the local authority will assess the amount that the resident has to pay towards the fees solely on the resident's income and savings. In England the *Health and Social Care Act 2008* repealed the 'liable relative' rule, which potentially required a spouse to contribute to care costs in a care home. The Welsh Assembly Government repealed the 'liable relative' rule in the Charges for Residential Accommodation CRAG amendment no. 25 issued 6 April 2009, Section IV. It had already been repealed in Scotland under Section 62 of the Adult Support and Protection (Scotland) Act 2000. An unmarried partner or civil partner has no liability under the local authority charging procedures to pay for a partner's care.

143

If you have an occupational or personal pension and your spouse is not living in a care home with you, the local authority will ignore half the pension when assessing your income if you pass at least this amount to your spouse. This rule also applies to civil partners.

The local authority can also use its discretion to vary the amount of the Personal Expenses Allowance. For example, you might want to ask for this to happen if you are not married to your partner, as the local authority will not automatically ignore half of your pension in this situation.

The person at home may be able to claim benefits such as Pension Credit in their own right, depending on their income and savings.

FOR MORE INFORMATION about paying for care in a care home in England and Wales if you have a partner, contact Age UK Advice on 0800 169 65 65. In Scotland, call the Scottish Helpline for Older People (SHOP) on 0845 125 9732. In Northern Ireland, call Age NI Advice on 0808 808 7575.

Attendance Allowance or Disability Living Allowance in a care home

The mobility component of DLA is not affected by admission to a care home unless you receive full funding from the NHS.

Whether or not you can receive AA or the care component of DLA will depend on how the fees are being met.

If you are paying the full charges in a care home, you can claim and receive AA or DLA care component provided you fulfil the other conditions (see pages 98–104). You can receive these allowances whether you arranged the admission yourself or the local authority arranged the admission. Payments for nursing care in a home providing nursing do not affect your ability to receive AA or DLA. In Scotland, if the local authority pays for your personal care costs, you cannot receive AA or the care component of DLA. If the NHS pays the full fees, your AA or DLA will be affected because you will normally be regarded as a hospital inpatient (see page 105).

If you need local authority financial support in order to meet the home's fees, you cannot start to receive AA or the care component of DLA. If you are already receiving one of these allowances, it will stop four weeks after the admission – or sooner if you have moved in from hospital.

However, you may retain an 'underlying entitlement' to the allowance, so that if, for example, you move out of the care home, you could start receiving it again without making a fresh claim. You should contact the DWP and ask for the allowance to be paid again. If the local authority temporarily provides funding but will later be reimbursed in full by you – for example, under a deferred payment agreement – AA or the care component of DLA can be paid for that period. Pension Credit can be paid at the same time as AA or the care component of DLA in these circumstances, although it may not be available if you own a house that is not being marketed. Get advice if your AA or DLA has been stopped and you do not think that it should have been.

FOR MORE INFORMATION, in England and Wales see the Age UK factsheet Paying for Permanent Residential Care *available from Age UK Advice on 0800 169 65 65. In Scotland, call the Scottish Helpline for Older People (SHOP) on 0845 125 9732. In Northern Ireland, call Age NI Advice on 0808 808 7575.*

The Care Quality Commission and standards in care homes

The regulation and maintenance of standards in care homes in England is carried out by the Care Quality Commission. It has a star rating system for registered care homes, based on its inspection regime. Impartial information about the quality of a particular care home can be obtained on its website (www.cqc.org.uk). If you are in a care home and you are concerned with the quality of care you are receiving, you can inform the Care Quality Commission, who must take appropriate action.

In Wales these responsibilities are carried out by the Care and Social Services Inspectorate Wales, which is based at CSSIW National Office, 4–5 Charnwood Court, Heol Billingsley, Nantgarw CF15 7QZ. Telephone: 01443 848450. Website: www.csiw.wales.gov.uk.

In Scotland these responsibilities are currently covered by the Scottish Commission for Regulation of Care (SCRC), otherwise known as the Care Commission. They are based regionally, but their headquarters are based at Compass House, Riverside Drive, Dundee DD1 4NY. Telephone: 01382 207 100; Helpline 0845 603 0890. Website: www.carecommission.com.

Human rights in care homes

The *Health and Social Care Act 2008* extended the protections contained in the *Human Rights Act 1998* to UK residents placed in independent care homes by a local authority. These protections were previously only available in local authority-run care homes.

Changes to the local authority and Ombudsman complaints procedure

If you are not satisfied with any aspect of the service being received from a local authority, you can make a complaint through its complaints procedure. Information on the procedure should be available on request. In April 2009 the existing local authority procedure was replaced by a unified health and social care complaints framework. You still have the right to take a complaint to the Local Government Ombudsman if you do not agree with the outcome of a complaint in England. In Wales you should refer to the Public Services Ombudsman for Wales. In Scotland you should refer to the Scottish Public Services Ombudsman (SPSO).

From October 2010 adults who fund their own social care, at home or in a care home, will have access to an independent complaints review service provided by the Local Government Ombudsman. This new right is included in the *Health Act 2009*.

Safeguarding older people from abuse

If you have any concerns related to the abuse of an older person in any circumstance, you can contact the local authority to discuss the issue. They will have a safeguarding adults policy, designed to respond appropriately to the various types of issues that are raised in this area.

Other Benefits and Financial Support

This part of *Your Rights* gives details about other benefits and financial help that may be available for older people. It covers Working Tax Credit and benefits for people who are unemployed or bereaved. It then describes other types of financial support and concessions, including help with paying for fuel and other household bills, health costs and travel concessions. There is also information about help with the Council Tax.

WORKING TAX CREDIT

Single people or couples who are employed or self-employed can claim Working Tax Credit. There is no upper age limit for making a claim. To qualify for Working Tax Credit you must normally be living in the UK and: if you qualify for the 'disability element' or the '50 plus element', you must work for at least 16 hours a week; or if you do not qualify for these elements, you must work for at least 30 hours a week and be over 25 years old.

From April 2011 people over 60 will be able to claim Working Tax Credit if they work for at least 16 hours a week.

To qualify for the 50 plus element you must be aged 50 or over and returning to work for at least 16 hours a week after coming off certain benefits. For the six months before you started work you should have been receiving at least one of the following benefits:

- State Pension together with Pension Credit;
- Jobseeker's Allowance (JSA);
- Incapacity Benefit;
- Employment and Support Allowance (ESA);
- Income Support;
- Carer's Allowance;
- Bereavement Allowance;
- Widowed Mother's Allowance;
- Severe Disablement Allowance;
- Training Allowance paid under the Work Based Learning for Adults or Training for Work schemes (in England, Wales and Scotland); or
- National Insurance (NI) credits; for example, because of unemployment, incapacity or caring responsibilities.

The 50 plus element is paid for only 12 months.

You may qualify for the disability element if you have a disability that puts you at a disadvantage in getting a job and if you are, or have recently been, receiving an incapacity or disability benefit including Incapacity Benefit, ESA, Disability Living Allowance (DLA) or Attendance Allowance (AA).

If you fulfil these criteria, whether you will receive Working Tax Credit, and if so how much, will depend on your circumstances and your income (including that of your partner if you have one).

Working Tax Credit is administered by HM Revenue & Customs (HMRC, formerly Inland Revenue) and the assessment of income and savings is done on a yearly basis. For the tax year 2010/11 any Working Tax Credit you receive will be an estimated amount based either on your previous year's income or on an estimate of your current income. Your award will only be finalised after April 2011 when your actual income for 2010/11 is known. If you have been underpaid tax credits, you will get the extra amount you are owed, but if you have been overpaid some tax credits, you may have to pay them back, usually by recovery from next year's award.

FOR MORE INFORMATION or a claim form, contact your local Jobcentre Plus office or Tax Enquiry Centre, or ring the Tax Credits Helpline on 0845 300 3900.

JOBSEEKER'S ALLOWANCE

JSA is a taxable benefit for people who are unemployed. There are two elements: contribution-based JSA, which is based on your NI contribution record, and income-based JSA, which is means-tested.

To qualify for JSA you must be:

* under State Pension age (although if you are a man who has reached Pension Credit qualifying age, see

page 46; you may be better off claiming Pension Credit than JSA);

- unemployed or working for fewer than 16 hours a week;
- capable of and available for work; and
- actively seeking work – you must have entered into a Jobseeker's Agreement and you must comply with any directions given.

Contribution-based JSA This can be paid for a maximum of 182 days (26 weeks) if you have paid enough NI contributions. The rate for people aged 25 or over is £65.45. There are no additions for dependants. If you have an occupational or personal pension of over £50 a week, this will reduce your contribution-based JSA by the amount by which your pension exceeds £50, although in general other income you may have and your savings are not taken into account.

Income-based JSA This can be paid in addition to the contribution-based JSA, or on its own if you do not have sufficient NI contributions or you have already received contribution-based JSA for 26 weeks. To qualify for income-based JSA you must have no more than £16,000 savings and be on a low income.

If you have a partner, their income and savings will be added to yours, and your partner must either not be in work or be working for fewer than 24 hours a week on average. Couples may be required to make a joint claim where both partners need to be actively seeking work and to have entered into a Jobseeker's Agreement. If your partner is over the woman's State Pension age or cannot work, for example because they are disabled or are a carer, or if they are working at least 16 hours a week but fewer than 24, they will not have to meet the job-seeking requirements.

The amount of income-based JSA you receive will vary according to your age, your other income and savings, and your entitlement to any premiums. Premiums are paid to people receiving certain disability benefits, to carers and to people with dependent children, for example. Homeowners may get some help with certain housing costs (such as mortgage interest).

When working out your benefit, most of your income is taken into account, but some income, such as DLA, is ignored. Any capital you have above £6,000 (or £10,000 if you or your partner is over the qualifying age for Pension Credit) will be assumed to produce a weekly income, which will also be taken into account when calculating the amount of your benefit.

If you qualify for income-based JSA, you may also get other benefits such as Housing Benefit and Council Tax Benefit and help with NHS costs.

You may be able to claim another benefit rather than JSA, depending on your circumstances. If you or your partner has reached the qualifying age for Pension Credit, you may be better off claiming Pension Credit. If you or your partner is incapable of work because of disability or illness, you may be able to claim ESA, or a person who is a carer may be able to claim Income Support.

How to claim

As soon as you need to look for work or need to claim benefit, you should phone Jobcentre Plus. In some areas, they will collect information over the phone and produce a statement of your circumstances for you to sign. This will mean that you might not have to complete certain claim forms. During the phone call, they will ask you about your situation, and what help you want. As well as offering help finding a job, they will arrange a meeting for you with a personal adviser, usually in a Jobcentre Plus office.

At the meeting, your adviser should discuss benefits and other support, as well as covering employment options. At

153

the end of the interview, you will have to sign a Jobseeker's Agreement that outlines the action you are expected to take to find work. Once JSA is awarded, you will need to attend your local office, usually every two weeks.

In some situations, JSA may not be paid for a limited period. For example, if the Jobcentre considers that you left work voluntarily without 'just cause' or if you refuse to take a job without 'good cause', you may lose benefit for up to 26 weeks. You can appeal against decisions to suspend your benefit. You may lose benefit if you accept early retirement, although not if you are made redundant.

FOR MORE INFORMATION if you are refused benefit or need help or advice with claiming JSA, contact a local advice agency.

INCOME SUPPORT AND INCOME-RELATED EMPLOYMENT AND SUPPORT ALLOWANCE

Income Support is a means-tested benefit based on your income and savings, and which is intended to help with basic weekly living costs. The information here applies to people who have not reached the qualifying age for Pension Credit – when you reach that age you may be able to get Pension Credit instead (see page 46). Income Support is paid to people who do not have to sign on for work – for example, people who are receiving Statutory Sick Pay (SSP) or who are carers or lone parents. If you are unable to work because of sickness or disability (and not receiving SSP) you should claim income-related ESA instead.

Income Support or income-related ESA can be paid on their own if you have no other income, or they can top up other benefits or part-time earnings. If you do not have much money coming in and have no more than £16,000 in savings, it is worth checking to see if you can qualify for Income Support or income-related ESA (though if you have reached the qualifying age for Pension Credit, you may be better off claiming that). If you have a partner, their income and savings will be added to yours. You cannot get Income Support or income-related ESA if you work 16 or more hours a week or if your partner works 24 or more hours a week (but see rules on 'permitted work' for ESA on page 120).

The amount of Income Support or income-related ESA you receive will vary according to your age, your other income and savings, and your entitlement to any premiums. Premiums are paid to people receiving certain disability benefits, to carers and to some people with dependent children. Homeowners may get some help with certain housing costs (such as mortgage interest). The rules are similar to those for Pension Credit, but there are some differences, so contact an advice organisation for more information.

When working out your benefit, most of your income is taken into account, but some income, such as DLA, is ignored. Any capital you have above £6,000 (or £10,000 if you or your partner is over the qualifying age for Pension Credit) will be assumed to produce a weekly income, which will also be taken into account when calculating the amount of your benefit.

Incapacity Benefit and Income Support paid on the grounds of incapacity have now been replaced by ESA. There are two elements to this benefit, contributory ESA (which is similar to Incapacity Benefit) and income-related ESA (which is similar to Income Support paid on the grounds of incapacity). ESA claimants are divided into two separate groups: the 'support group' and the 'work-related activity group'. The group you are placed in will determine how much you are paid and the responsibilities you will need to meet in order to keep receiving the benefit.

In order to qualify for income-related ESA you must meet all of the following conditions:

- have a limited capacity for work;
- not be in work;
- be aged 16 or over;
- be under State Pension age (65 for men; see Chapter 1 for a how a woman's State Pension age is calculated);
- be in Great Britain;
- not be entitled to Income Support;
- not be entitled to JSA (and not a member of a couple entitled to joint-claim JSA); and
- not be within a period of entitlement to Statutory Sick Pay.

You must also meet at least one of the following conditions:

- you satisfy the NI contribution requirements; or
- your limited capability for work began before you were 20 (or 25 in some cases); or
- you satisfy the conditions for income-related ESA.

You can be entitled to both contributory ESA and income-related ESA at the same time.

To claim Income Support or ESA, contact your local Jobcentre Plus office. If you need more advice about Income Support or ESA, contact a local advice agency.

BEREAVEMENT BENEFITS

Bereavement Benefits are generally available to men and women under State Pension age when their husband, wife or civil partner dies. Entitlement is based on the National Insurance contribution record of the person who has died. Information given in this section covers the Bereavement Payment and the Bereavement Allowance. There is also a Widowed Parent's Allowance for people with dependent children.

FOR MORE INFORMATION on Bereavement Benefits, contact a local advice agency or Jobcentre Plus office. Or you can telephone 0845 608 8602 if you live in Scotland, North-West England or East of England; 0845 608 8601 if you live in any other area.

When you register a death, the Registrar will give you Form BD8 (Form 344S1 in Scotland) to send to your local Jobcentre Plus or pension centre. If you wish to claim Bereavement Benefits, answer 'yes' to the appropriate question on the reverse of the form.

People over State Pension age whose husband, wife or civil partner dies may be entitled to claim a State Pension based on their late partner's contributions, as explained on pages 9–11.

Women widowed before 9 April 2001 may be receiving Widow's Pension (see pages 158–159).

Any earnings you receive will not affect your Bereavement Benefits, Widow's Pension or State Pension.

Bereavement Payment

The Bereavement Payment is a single lump-sum payment of £2,000. It is tax-free and is paid mainly to widows, widowers and surviving civil partners under State Pension age. Entitlement depends on the NI contributions of the deceased at the date of their death . If you are over State Pension age when your husband, wife or civil partner dies, you can qualify for a payment if:

- your partner was under State Pension age when they died; or
- your partner was over State Pension age when they died but not entitled to a State Pension based on their own contribution record (for example, if your wife was over State Pension age when she died and she received a State Pension based on your contributions).

Bereavement Allowance

The Bereavement Allowance is paid to both men and women who are aged at least 45 but under State Pension age when they are bereaved and whose husband, wife or civil partner fulfilled the NI contribution conditions. The full standard rate of £97.65 is paid if you are aged 55 or over when you are bereaved. If you are aged 45 to 54, you will receive a percentage of the standard rate. You cannot receive any of your partner's Additional State Pension.

Bereavement Allowance will be paid for a maximum of 52 weeks but will stop if during that period you:

- remarry;
- form a civil partnership;
- live with someone as though you were married or civil partners; or
- reach State Pension age.

Once you reach State Pension age you may be able to claim a State Pension based on your late husband, wife or civil partner's contributions, as explained on pages 9–11.

Widow's Pension

If your husband died before 9 April 2001, you may be in receipt of a Widow's Pension and this will not have been affected by the introduction of Bereavement Benefits. The full standard rate is £97.65, but you may be getting less if you were between 40 and 49 when you were widowed.

You may also be receiving an additional State Pension based on your husband's earnings since 1978, taking into account any periods that he was a member of a contracted-out occupational pension scheme or personal pension scheme.

When you reach State Pension age (see Chapter 1 for more details of the women's State Pension age), you can claim the State Pension instead of the Widow's Pension or you can remain on the Widow's Pension until you reach 65. The amounts will often be the same, but you may also receive some Graduated Retirement Benefit with the State Pension. Check with the DWP what the different amounts would be.

The Widow's Pension will not be affected by your earnings. However, if you do not claim your State Pension when you reach the qualifying age, you will not earn extra State Pension unless you give up the Widow's Pension (see page 28 on deferring your penson). If you remarry or form a civil partnership before you reach the State Pension age, you will lose the Widow's Pension. It will also be suspended during any period when you live with someone as their partner. However, if you are State Pension age or over and receive a State Pension based on your previous husband's contributions, you will not lose this if you remarry or live with someone as though you were married or civil partners.

FOR MORE INFORMATION, see DWP guide NP45 A guide to Bereavement Benefits, which is available only on the website (www.dwp.gov.uk), and Jobcentre Plus leaflet WIDA5 If you are widowed or your civil partner dies.

HOUSEHOLD BILLS, INSULATION AND REPAIRS

This section looks at some of the main household bills and expenses that older people face. It briefly covers dealing with debt and then summarises the help that may be available for different expenses, referring you to Age UK factsheets and other sources where appropriate. More detailed information is given about:

- paying for fuel and insulation;
- help with repairs;
- the Council Tax.

Debt problems

Many older people have to manage on low incomes and sometimes face particular problems when an unexpected bill comes in or income drops because of a change in circumstances, such as divorce or bereavement. If you are having difficulty managing, check to see whether you are entitled to any additional income such as the benefits described in this book (for example, Pension Credit, Housing Benefit or Council Tax Benefit). Then write down the amount of money you need for essential everyday living. This should help you to work out a statement of income and expenditure, which you can then use to negotiate smaller payments to your creditors.

Many people underestimate their basic living expenses and then try to pay their bills at a higher rate than they can really afford. Once they see the reality of your situation, most creditors should freeze interest and accept payments that you can afford.

If this seems too much to have to deal with, seek advice. There are many independent advice agencies that can help with debt problems, including Citizens Advice, or you can ring National Debtline on 0808 808 4000 (free call).

FOR MORE INFORMATION, see the Age UK factsheet Debt Management, *which is available from Age UK Advice on 0800 169 65 65.*

Help with bills and expenses

Fuel There are no regular, weekly social security payments towards fuel bills but there are Winter Fuel Payments and Cold Weather Payments, as described below. Grants towards insulation and draught-proofing may help you heat your home more effectively. Some fuel companies have charitable trusts to help vulnerable customers with fuel debts. Help is discretionary and criteria for eligibility are set by individual companies.

Rent and mortgage costs Means-tested help towards rent comes through Housing Benefit (see pages 70–90), while homeowners may get help with their mortgage interest payments and certain service charges through Pension Credit (see pages 46–70) or Income Support, income-related ESA, or income-based JSA if aged under Pension Credit qualifying age (see page 151).

Council Tax Council Tax Benefit (see pages 70–90) is means-tested. There are also other ways of reducing Council Tax bills, which are described on pages 174.

Water charges There are no social security benefits to help with the cost of water or sewerage charges. Some water companies have charitable trusts to help vulnerable customers with water debts. Help is discretionary and criteria for eligibility are set by individual companies. Some customers may be able to get help with the costs of water supply under the Vulnerable Groups Scheme (WaterSure). This scheme is open to people who are receiving certain qualifying benefits and who have water meters and use a high volume of water because of certain medical conditions, or because they have three or more children under the age of 19 and in full-time education living in the property. Contact your water company for more information.

FOR MORE INFORMATION see Age UK Factsheet 69 Water Advice.

The system is different in Scotland and Northern Ireland. There is only one supplier of water and sewerage services in Scotland – Scottish Water. The one water supplier in Northern Ireland is Northern Ireland Water.

FOR MORE INFORMATION on services in Scotland, contact Scottish Water on 0845 601 8855 (for emergencies 0845 600 8855) or contact the Scottish Helpline for Older People (SHOP) on 0845 125 9732. For Northern Ireland, contact Northern Ireland Water on 028 90 244711.

Telephone costs   There is no national scheme providing financial help with phone charges. Some people who are ill or disabled may be able to receive help from their local authority social services department. This help could include a payment to cover the installation costs of the phone and sometimes the rental costs. The local authority may also help with aids and adaptations to the phone; for example, lamp signalling handsets for people with hearing difficulties. If you have been on Pension Credit, Income Support, income-based JSA or income-related ESA for at least 26 weeks, you may be able to get a loan from the Social Fund (see pages 90–95) to cover the cost of installing a phone.

BT offers a low-cost line-rental scheme that is available to customers who receive one of the following benefits: Income Support, income-based JSA, Pension Credit Guarantee Credit or income-related ESA. For more information contact BT.

Repairs, improvements and adaptations   In some situations you may be able to receive a grant to help with household repairs, adaptations or improvements, as explained on pages 171–174.

PAYING FOR FUEL AND INSULATION

The cost of fuel is a major expense for most pensioners. This section outlines what help is available.

Fuel debts

If you are threatened with disconnection because you cannot pay your bills, contact your energy supplier straight away. You may be able to agree a repayment plan to pay your arrears or have a pre-payment meter installed.

If you have a fuel debt and are receiving Pension Credit, Income Support, income-related ESA or income-based JSA you may be able to avoid disconnection or get reconnected by going onto the Third Party Deductions Scheme. Some of your benefit will be withheld every week and paid direct to the company. The scheme covers the following essential household bills as well:

- housing costs;
- rent arrears, service charges for heating, lighting;
- water charges (water, then sewerage, if there are two debts);
- Council Tax and community charge arrears;
- fines;
- Child Support maintenance under the old scheme;
- integration loans;
- eligible loans.

Suppliers are not allowed to disconnect supplies for non-payment of bills (provided this is not deliberate) during winter months to households where all the occupants are pensioners.

Social tariffs

Energy providers may offer social tariffs to consumers who are having difficulty paying their bills. The criteria of eligibility are different for different suppliers. All social tariffs should equal the suppliers' cheapest deals but some customers may still be better off by switching to another supplier.

FOR MORE INFORMATION, see the Consumer Focus website (www.consumerfocus.org.uk) or talk to Consumer Direct on 08454 040506. For details of currently available social tariffs, contact your supplier.

Energy Rebate Scheme

In 2010 you may be entitled to a one-off rebate of £80 on your electricity bill under the energy rebate scheme that the Government has arranged with some electricity suppliers. You may be eligible if you were aged 70 or over on 26 March 2010, you are responsible for the electricity account where you live and you are receiving the guarantee part of Pension Credit only (that is, you are not receiving savings credit). The rebate will not be given to people getting some social tariffs. You must also be a customer of one of the participating electricity suppliers. To find out which suppliers participate in the scheme go to the Direct Gov website (www.direct.gov.uk).

If you are eligible, you should receive a letter by the end of June 2010 and the payment should be credited automatically to your electricity account.

FOR MORE INFORMATION, contact the Energy Rebate Scheme helpline on 0845 600 0033.

Priority services

All gas and electricity suppliers must offer special services to people of pensionable age and people who have a disability or a long-term illness. These services include the following:

- You are entitled to a free annual safety check for gas appliances and installations if you are a homeowner and you receive means-tested benefits, and either all adults in the household are eligible for free services or the household includes a child under five years old.
- You can request a quarterly meter reading if no one in the house can read the meter. A password is provided so that you can confirm the identity of the electricity or gas supplier employee calling at your home.
- You can request that your bill is sent to a nominated third party if you find bills difficult to read or understand.
- There is a priority service for getting your gas supply restored or, if necessary, arranging temporary heating and cooking facilities, provided that all adults living in your home are eligible for the priority services.

For more information and to register, contact your gas or electricity supplier.

Winter Fuel Payments

Winter Fuel Payments provide help with the cost of fuel bills for pensioner households. They are paid to most people who have reached women's State Pension age, which is increasing from 60 to 65 between April 2010 and April 2020 (see page 3). There are no income or savings limits, and they are not taxable. The payments for each year are based on someone's age during the qualifying week in that year, which is normally the week beginning the third Monday in September. To be eligible for a payment in winter 2010/11 on the grounds of your age you will need to have been born on or before 5 July 1950.

The Winter Fuel Payment is normally £200 and £300 where someone in the household is aged 80 or over. The Winter Fuel Payment for 2010/11 is expected to include an extra £50 for 60–79-year-olds and £100 for households with someone aged 80 or over, making the payments £250 and £400 respectively.

> *FOR DETAILS of what payment you can expect, or to make a claim, contact the Winter Fuel Helpline on 0845 915 1515.*

Although payments are normally made only to people living in the UK, some people who qualify for a Winter Fuel Payment in the UK and move to another European Economic Area (EEA) country or Switzerland may be able to continue to receive payments.

> *FOR MORE INFORMATION on this specific issue, ring the Winter Fuel Team at the International Pension Centre, on 0191 218 7777.*

Cold Weather Payments

If you receive Pension Credit, Income Support, income-based JSA or income-related ESA, you may be eligible for Cold Weather Payments. If you are receiving Income Support or income-based JSA, this must include a pensioner or disability premium or there must be a child under five years old. A payment is made when the average temperature at a specified weather station has been recorded as, or is forecast to be, 0° Celsius or below over seven consecutive days. The rate for 2010/11 is £25.00 for each week of cold weather. Savings are not taken into account. These payments will be made automatically, so you do not have to make a claim.

Grants for energy efficiency

If you live in England   Warm Front is a government-funded scheme set up to provide energy advice and grants to improve home energy efficiency. It is available to certain groups of people who own or privately rent their home and who are in receipt of qualifying benefits.

The Warm Front provides a package of energy efficient insulation and heating measures tailored to each property, up to the value of £3,500 (or up to the value of £6,000 for those in areas without gas supply). It may include gas, electric or oil-fired central heating, cavity and loft insulation, draught-proofing, hot-water-tank insulation, converting a solid-fuel open fire to a modern glass-fronted fire, energy efficiency advice and low-energy light bulbs.

Households that have already received assistance from Warm Front are able to apply for additional measures. The value of the grant available to properties previously helped will be the balance of £3,500 (or £6,000 for those in areas without gas supply) less the value of all works completed since June 2000.

166

The Warm Front grant is available to householders who are State Pension age or over and in receipt of Pension Credit, Housing Benefit, Council Tax Benefit, Income Support, income-based JSA or income-related ESA. It is also available to those who have young children or who are disabled and receive qualifying income-related or disability-related benefits. Householders whose spouse, civil partner or partner fulfils the eligibility criteria are also eligible. A partner means a person with whom the applicant lives as if they were husband and wife, or a civil partner.

The Warm Front schemes are being promoted and run by the Eaga Partnership Ltd, the managing organisation appointed by the Government. Eaga will arrange for a surveyor to visit and assess what work needs to be done. In rented accommodation the landlord's consent is needed before any work can be undertaken. Landlords must not put rent up because of the improvements funded by the Warm Front for a set period (one year following insulation works or two years following heating works).

Householders who are State Pension age or over and are not entitled to the Warm Front Grant can receive a grant up to a maximum of £300 (the Heating Rebate) for the provision or replacement of certain heating systems. Qualifying applicants will have to use one of the installers approved by Eaga and the payment will be made directly to the installer on completion of the work.

FOR MORE INFORMATION see Age UK Factsheet 1 Help with Heating Costs *or Factsheet 1w* Help with Heating in Wales. *You can also contact Age UK Advice on 0800 169 65 65 or Warm Front on 0800 316 2805, or go to the Warm Front website (www.warmfront.co.uk).*

If you live in Wales The Home Energy Efficiency Scheme in Wales (HEES Wales) provides grants for people of State Pension age or over who are receiving one of the following income-related benefits: Pension Credit, Housing Benefit, Council Tax Benefit, income-based JSA, or certain disability benefits, including DLA and AA. People over 80 also qualify automatically. The grant may offer a variety of insulation measures, including cavity wall/loft insulation, draught-proofing and a range of heating improvements, including the installation of gas or electric central heating for those without central heating, the conversion of an existing solid-fuel system, repairs to systems that are not working, energy efficiency advice, smoke alarms and a benefit entitlement check. If you are State Pension age or over, own your home and are not on any benefit, you may be eligible for a 25% grant towards the cost of the above measures up to £500. Other householders may also qualify for the scheme as eligibility varies; contact your local Energy Efficiency Advice Centre on 0800 512 012 or visit the Energy Saving Trust website (www.energysavingtrust.org.uk).

If you live in Scotland   In Scotland energy efficiency grants are made under the Energy Assistance Package (formerly known as the Central Heating and Warm Deal schemes). The grant covers a package of energy efficiency measures, all or some of which may be offered, according to the energy needs of the home. The package has four stages:

- **Stage 1** offers free expert energy advice to anyone who phones the Energy Savings Scotland advice centre (ESSAC) network on 0800 512 012.
- **Stage 2** provides benefits and tax credit checks and advice on low-cost energy tariffs to those at risk of fuel poverty.
- **Stage 3** provides a package of standard insulation measures (cavity wall and loft insulation) to older households and those on one of a range of benefits. If you are a private tenant, you may qualify for a package of standard insulation measures (cavity

wall and loft insulation) if you are a homeowner or the tenant of a private landlord and you or your partner:

○ is aged 70 or over and you have no central heating; or

○ is aged 75 or over; or

○ is receive a qualifying benefit.

If you are a social tenant, renting from either a local authority or Registered Social Landlord, similar insulation measures may be available to you funded through a partnership between your landlord, the Scottish Government and energy companies. For information about this you should contact your landlord.

• **Stage 4** offers a package of enhanced energy efficiency measures to those who are most vulnerable to fuel poverty. You may qualify for enhanced measures if you are a homeowner or the tenant of a private sector landlord and you or your partner:

○ is aged 60 or over and have no central heating system in your home;

○ you live in an energy inefficient home and you or your partner:

  □ is aged 75 or over;

  □ is aged 60 or over and receives a qualifying benefit;

  □ has a child under five years old and receives a qualifying benefit;

  □ has a disabled child under 16 years old and receives a qualifying benefit;

  □ is pregnant and receives a qualifying benefit.

Qualifying benefits include the following;

○ Attendance Allowance;

○ Child Tax Credit – where income less than £17,474;

- Council Tax Benefit;
- Housing Benefit;
- Income Support;
- income-based JSA;
- DLA;
- disablement pension that includes a Constant Attendance Allowance;
- State Pension Credit – with Guarantee Credit element;
- War Disablement Pension that includes a mobility supplement or a Constant Attendance Allowance;
- Working Tax Credit – where income less than £17,474;
- ESA.

The Energy Saving Trust manages delivery of the package on behalf of the Scottish Government.

FOR MORE INFORMATION about what the package can offer you, telephone the Energy Saving Trust on 0800 512 012 or go to the website (www.energyassistancepackage.com). For general information about the scheme, phone the Scottish Helpline for Older People (SHOP) on 0845 125 9732.

Help with energy efficiency from energy suppliers

If you are aged 70 or over or receiving certain benefits and live in private rented accommodation or you are an owner-occupier, you may be able to get free cavity wall and/or loft insulation. If you are not in one of these categories, you may be able to get a 50% discount on the above insulation measures.

FOR MORE INFORMATION, contact your local Energy Efficiency Advice Centre on 0800 512 012. Your local council or your energy provider should also be able to advise you further.

HELP WITH REPAIRS, IMPROVEMENTS AND ADAPTATIONS

England and Wales

Local authorities (councils) have general powers to provide assistance for repairs, improvements and adaptations to housing.

The assistance provided by the local authority may be provided in any form, including loans, grants, labour, materials or advice. It might be provided unconditionally, or subject to conditions such as repayment of all or part of the assistance or a contribution towards the work for which assistance is required. The local authority must publish a policy, setting out the type of assistance it will provide and in what circumstances. It should also tell you how to make an enquiry and apply for assistance. A summary of the policy must be available to the public on request.

Local authorities also provide disabled facilities grants (DFG), which are mandatory in specific circumstances. A grant must be given if you are disabled and do not have access to your home and to the basic amenities within it (such as a bathroom, toilet or kitchen), provided that you qualify on income grounds – the grants are means-tested (but not if they are made in respect of disabled children). If you receive Pension Credit Guarantee Credit, Income Support or income-based JSA, Housing Benefit, Council Tax Benefit or Working Tax Credits or Child Tax Credit with gross taxable income of less than £15,050, you will not normally have to make a contribution. From 5 August 2009, income-related ESA has been also included as a passporting benefit.

FOR MORE INFORMATION, contact the local authority or other agency, such as a local Age UK/Age Concern*,

*Many local Age Concerns are changing their name to Age UK.

because the system is complicated. A step-by-step guide on how to work out your contribution is included in the Disability Rights Handbook *(see page 206).*

The formal application for the grant must be made to the housing department of the local authority. The housing department must consult with the social services department to decide if the adaptations are necessary and appropriate. This will normally mean that you will receive a visit from an occupational therapist from social services to assess your needs and make recommendations on what work needs to be done.

The maximum amount for a mandatory disabled facilities grant is £30,000 in England and £36,000 in Wales.

In addition, local authorities are able to give discretionary assistance for adaptations or to help the occupant to move to alternative, more suitable, accommodation. There is no restriction on the amount of assistance that may be given. It may be paid in addition, or as an alternative, to the grant. You should not start the work or buy any of the materials until you have received the local authority's approval to go ahead.

In England, minor adaptations costing less than £1,000, and equipment that helps disabled people to manage daily tasks around the home, are required to be provided free of charge to those who are eligible.

If you receive Pension Credit, Income Support or income-based JSA or income-related ESA you may be able to claim a discretionary Community Care Grant or Budgeting Loan for minor household repairs (see pages 91–92).

In some areas there are Home Improvement Agencies (sometimes called Care and Repair or Staying Put projects) that provide support for vulnerable people, such as older people or disabled people, who are homeowners or who live in private rented accommodation, to help them undertake repairs, improvements or adaptations to their home. Your local authority or local Age UK/Age Concern* should know whether there is a scheme in your area, or you can contact Foundations, the national coordinating body for Home Improvement Agencies, at the address on pages 207-208.

FOR MORE INFORMATION see Age UK Factsheet 13 Funding Repairs, Improvements and Adaptations. *You can also contact Age UK Advice on 0800 169 65 65.*

Scotland

In Scotland the system of grants is different and only brief information is given here. Grants were available from the local authority housing department to owners and, in certain circumstances, private tenants to help meet the cost of improvement and repair work. The amount of grant you received depended on your financial circumstances, but in some cases a minimum grant of 50% was available. However, from April 2010 the system is changing, with local authorities introducing a new 'scheme of assistance' offering advice and help to people who need to carry out repair and improvement work to their homes. The new scheme aims to help more people keep their homes in good condition than the current scheme, by offering a wider range of services. Rather than focusing solely on financial help, under the new scheme councils will offer advice, practical assistance and, in some situations, loans. Although grants for repairs and improvements will still be available, these will only be offered in fairly limited circumstances. You may also get help towards the costs of housing aids and adaptations if you are assessed by the local authority housing department as needing these. Some Care and Repair schemes may be able to help you through the process of applying for assistance.

*Many local Age Concerns are changing their name to Age UK.

FOR DETAILS OF GRANTS, or to find out about Care and Repair in your area, contact your local authority housing department or the Scottish Helpline for Older People (SHOP) on 0845 125 9732 or see Age Scotland's Factsheet 13s Older Homeowners: Financial Help with Repairs and Adaptations.

HELP WITH THE COUNCIL TAX

Council Tax is the system of paying towards local government services in England, Scotland and Wales. The rates system continues in Northern Ireland, with a new Rate Relief Scheme for people with incomes just outside the limit for Housing Benefit or who are getting only partial help with their rates.

Under the Council Tax system all domestic dwellings are allocated to one of eight bands (A–H), depending on their estimated value in April 1991. The level of tax for a property in band H will be three times as high as the tax for a property in band A. The banding system in Wales has changed to nine bands (A–I), based on property values in April 2003.

One bill will be sent to each household. One or more people will be legally responsible for paying the bill, although the household can choose how to divide up the bill.

Reducing your bill

There are various ways that your Council Tax bill may be reduced and these are summarised below. It may be possible to receive help from more than one of these schemes.

Exemptions Some properties, mainly certain empty ones, will be exempt, which means that there will be no Council Tax to pay. For example, your former home will be exempt if it is empty because you are living in a hospital or care home, or because you have gone to live with someone else in order to receive or provide personal care. A property is also exempt if a 'severely mentally impaired' person lives there alone and would be liable to pay the tax.

Disability reduction scheme   The property may be placed in a lower band if it has certain features that are important for a disabled person, such as extra space for a wheelchair or an additional bathroom or kitchen for the use of the disabled person. If your home qualifies for a reduction, your bill will be reduced to the level of tax for the band below the one your home is in. Since April 2000, properties in the lowest band (A) that have the relevant disability features have also qualified for a reduction. In this situation bills will be reduced by one-sixth. Contact your local authority if you think that your property would qualify for a reduction.

Discounts   The Council Tax rules assume that there are two or more people living in each property. A discount of a quarter (25%) will be given if someone lives alone and a discount of half (50%) will normally be given if no one is living there. Some people will not be counted for the purposes of the Council Tax, so discounts may still be given even if there are two or more people in a property. For example, someone who is 'severely mentally impaired' will not be counted. The discount can also apply to a carer who lives with and, for at least 35 hours a week, is caring for someone receiving the highest care component of DLA or the higher rate of AA. You will not be able to get this discount if the person you care for is your partner or is a child under 18.

Council Tax Benefit   This depends on the income and savings of the person(s) responsible for the bill or the people they live with. It is described in more detail on pages 70–90.

FOR MORE INFORMATION, contact Age UK Advice on 0800 169 65 65.

Lone Pensioner Allowance   A discount is available in Northern Ireland to help pay the rates; this is called the Lone Pensioner Allowance (LPA). You will be entitled to a 20% discount on your rates if you are a pensioner aged 70 or over, living on your own and paying rates for your home. The LPA is not means-tested. To apply phone 08448 920902 for more information or go to the website (www.helpwithratesni.gov.uk) and download an application form.

HELP WITH HEALTH COSTS

Most NHS treatment is free, but for some NHS services, you may have to pay part or all of the cost. This section first outlines hearing and chiropody services that may be free and then explains who can get help with the cost of NHS services you would normally be charged for, such as dental care, eye tests and glasses.

Free NHS services

Hearing aids   You should discuss hearing difficulties with your GP, who may, if necessary, refer you to the local hospital for tests. If you are prescribed a hearing aid for one or both ears, this will be fitted and issued by a local NHS hearing aid centre. NHS hearing aids are available on free loan; repairs and batteries are also free. It is possible to buy hearing aids from a private company, but these can be expensive and are not necessarily more effective.

> FOR MORE INFORMATION, contact the Royal National Institute for Deaf People (address on page 209), which publishes a range of information leaflets on hearing loss, hearing aids (including digital hearing aids) and other matters concerning deafness.

Chiropody/podiatry   NHS chiropody services (sometimes called podiatry services) are free if you have a medical foot problem or a health condition such as diabetes that puts you at risk of foot-related problems. In many areas, there are eligibility criteria that you must meet in order to be treated by a chiropodist as an NHS patient. Your GP or Primary Care Trust should be able to advise you about local NHS chiropody/podiatry services.

In some parts of the country, chiropody services are liaising with voluntary organisations, such as Age UK, to provide simple nail-cutting services and education in foot care to prevent problems. Contact Age UK Advice on 0800 169 65 65 for details of your nearest Age UK/Age Concern*. Contact them to see if they offer this service and whether there is a charge.

If you wish to consider private treatment, your local NHS chiropody department may have details of private practitioners. Alternatively, you could refer to Yellow Pages or go to the website of the Society of Chiropodists and Podiatrists (www.feetforlife.org). Make sure that the chiropodist is registered with the Health Professions Council (www.hpc-uk.org).

Help with NHS costs – NHS Low Income Scheme

If you (or your partner if you have one, and any dependent young person under 20 is included in the award) receive Pension Credit Guarantee Credit (with or without Pension Credit Savings Credit), Income Support, income-related JSA or income-related ESA (with or without contribution-based ESA), you are entitled to receive full help with the health costs described below by showing your award letter from the DWP. If you receive Working Tax Credit with Child Tax Credit or with a disability element (check your award letter), you may also get this help, but it will depend on your income. In the following paragraphs, wherever Pension Credit Guarantee Credit or Income Support are mentioned,

*Many local Age Concerns are changing their name to Age UK.

the above benefits are covered too. In certain circumstances help may also be available if you receive a War Pension.

On their own, contribution-based JSA, Pension Credit Savings Credit or contribution-based ESA do not entitle you to help with health costs.

If you do not receive one of the benefits mentioned above but are on a low income and have no more than £16,000 in savings, you can apply for help with costs of NHS dental treatment, glasses or contact lenses, and some travel costs incurred to receive NHS treatment, through the NHS Low Income Scheme. (The savings limit for people living permanently in care homes is different – £23,250.)

If you qualify for help with health costs, you will be sent one of two certificates. Certificate HC2 entitles you to full help with health costs, including free prescriptions, dental treatment, sight tests, full voucher value towards the cost of glasses and certain travel costs to receive NHS treatment. If your income is higher, you may get certificate HC3, which entitles you to partial help with these costs. The HC3 does not entitle you to any help with prescription charges if you would normally pay.

If you are single and over 65, or one of a couple where at least one of you is over 65, and your only income is state-benefit related, your HC2 or HC3 certificate will usually be awarded for five years; otherwise a certificate will be awarded for one year.

To apply for a certificate you will need to complete the form HC1. This is available if you ask at a Jobcentre Plus office or by phoning 0845 610 1112 or your local NHS hospital; some dentists, opticians and GP surgeries might also have them. (If you live permanently in a care home and receive financial support from the local authority, ask the owner or manager of the home for form HC1 (SC).) It is best to apply in advance. Remember that, if you receive Pension Credit Guarantee Credit, you do not need to apply for a certificate to receive help with these costs.

FOR MORE INFORMATION, see the Department of Health leaflet HC11 Help with health costs *or the Age UK Factsheet 61* Help with Health Costs *(which is available from Age UK Advice on 0800 169 65 65).*

Prescriptions   In England NHS prescriptions are currently free to people aged 60 or over. Younger adults can also get free prescriptions if they have a low income and limited savings or suffer from a 'specified medical condition' (these conditions are listed in leaflet HC11) and hold an exemption certificate.

The State Pension age for women (currently 60) will rise gradually from April 2010 until it is equalised with the male State Pension age (65) in April 2020. The Government recently announced that eligibility for pensioner benefits (for men and women), such as free prescriptions, will increase in line with the female State Pension age. No one currently receiving these benefits will be affected and there was no change to the age exemption criteria for free prescriptions in April 2010.

If you are under the qualifying age and your partner receives Pension Credit Guarantee Credit or Pension Credit Guarantee Credit with Savings Credit, your prescriptions are free. Any young person included in a Pension Credit Guarantee Credit award is entitled too. If you have a valid certificate HC2, as described above, anyone named on the certificate will be entitled to free prescriptions. People who have a valid certificate HC3 entitling them to partial help with some NHS costs cannot get free prescriptions.

If you cannot get free prescriptions but require regular prescriptions, you may be able to save money by buying a prescription pre-payment certificate (PPC) for either three or 12 months. A 12-month PPC can be purchased by 10 monthly direct debit payments or a lump sum payment.

FOR MORE INFORMATION about the PPC scheme or to request an application form (FP95), you can ring 0845 850 00 30. The form is also available from pharmacists. Your pharmacist can help you decide whether a PPC would be financially advantageous for you.

In Wales, prescriptions have been free for everyone since April 2007 and in Northern Ireland since April 2010.

In Scotland prescription charges are being phased out: charges from April 2009 were £4.00 (PPC £38.00 for 12 months), with a further reduction in April 2010 to £3.00 (PPC £28.00 for 12 months). They will be phased out completely in April 2011.

In Northern Ireland prescription charges have been free since April 2010.

Dental care   NHS dental treatment, check-ups and dentures are free if you or your partner get Pension Credit Guarantee Credit or if you have certificate HC2. The cost may be reduced if you have certificate HC3. Details of how to apply for a certificate are given above. Every time you start a new course of treatment, tell the dentist that you are on Pension Credit Guarantee Credit or have certificate HC2 or HC3. You will need to confirm your entitlement by showing your award letter or HC2/HC3 certificate.

In Wales, dental checks are free for all people over the age of 60 (this is not currently linked to State Pension age).

In Northern Ireland, unless you are entitled to free treatment or help with the cost of your treatment, you are required to pay 80% of the gross cost of the treatments up to a maximum of £384.

In Scotland, check-ups and dental examinations on the NHS are free of charge. Unless you are entitled to free treatment, or at least some help with the cost of treatment, there is a sliding scale of charges, starting at

£10.10 for a scale and polish, up to £139.04 for a full set of dentures.

The NHS operates a three-band system of patient charging per course of treatment in England and Wales. Unless you are entitled to free treatment or help with the cost of treatment, in England you will pay either £16.50 (Band 1), £45.60 (Band 2) or £198.00 (Band 3), depending on which band the most expensive part of your treatment falls into. In Wales, the bands are £12 (Band 1), £39 (Band 2) or £177 (Band 3).

> FOR MORE INFORMATION about which local dentists are offering NHS treatment, contact NHS Direct on 0845 46 47 if you live in England, or go to the NHS Choices website (www.nhs.uk). In Wales, go to the Health of Wales Information website (www.wales.nhs.uk). In Scotland, call the NHS Helpline on 0800 22 44 88 (please note this is not an emergency dental service) or call the Scottish Helpline for Older People (SHOP) on 0845 125 9732. In Northern Ireland go to the NI Direct website (www.nidirect.gov.uk).

No help is given towards the cost of private dental treatment. If you want NHS dental care, make sure that the dentist is providing you with NHS treatment before you start each course of treatment. You can do this when you discuss the proposed treatment with your dentist.

Sight tests and glasses   NHS-funded sight tests to check your vision and eye health are available to all people aged 60 or over. There is no definition of what an NHS sight test should include. Tests for conditions such as glaucoma and other eye diseases that are more likely in older people are particularly important, so always ask what tests will be included in your sight test. It is recommended that younger adults have a sight test every two years and those aged 70 and over have one every 12 months.

If you are under the qualifying age and your partner receives Pension Credit Guarantee Credit or Pension Credit

Guarantee Credit with Savings Credit you are entitled to an NHS-funded sight test. Any young person included in a Pension Credit Guarantee Credit award is entitled too. If you have a valid certificate HC2, as described above, you qualify for an NHS-funded sight test. NHS-funded sight tests are also available if you are in a priority group, which includes registered blind and partially sighted people, those who need complex lenses, and diagnosed diabetics. A person who has glaucoma or is considered to be at risk of glaucoma, or someone aged 40 or over who is the parent, brother, sister or son or daughter of a person with diagnosed glaucoma, also qualifies for NHS-funded sight tests.

If, for health reasons, you cannot get to the opticians for a sight test, you may be able to arrange for an optometrist to visit you at home. If you are entitled to an NHS-funded sight test, you will not have to pay for the visit. The Patient Advice and Liaison Service (PALS) for your local Primary Care Trust can tell you which local opticians offer home visits. Call NHS Direct on 0845 4647 for your PALS contact details.

You are entitled to a voucher towards the cost of glasses if you or your partner get Pension Credit Guarantee Credit or Pension Credit Guarantee Credit with Savings Credit, or have certificate HC2. You may get some help if you have certificate HC3. You may be able to claim a refund in some circumstances if you do not receive your certificate in time, but it is better to apply well in advance. If you require two different pairs of glasses – one for reading, one for distance – you are entitled to two vouchers.

The voucher carries a financial value linked to your optical prescription; it may cover the full cost of the glasses or be used as part-payment for a more expensive pair. If your glasses or contact lenses cost more than any voucher you are given, you will have to pay the difference. If you need complex lenses, your optician can give you a voucher to help pay for the glasses regardless of your income and savings. However, the amount of help will be greater if you or your partner receive Pension Credit Guarantee Credit or qualify on the grounds of low income.

You do not have to get your glasses from the optometrist who carries out your sight test. If you prefer to go to a different optician, simply take your prescription with you and any voucher you are entitled to. If you have to pay some or all of the cost, it is best to 'shop around' to check whether another optician might be cheaper, as charges can vary.

If you have a serious eye condition or require specialist hospital care, you pay up to a maximum charge and the hospital meets the difference between the maximum charge and the cost of the glasses.

FOR MORE INFORMATION on eye problems and NHS-funded sight tests, contact the Royal National Institute of Blind People at the address on page 209.

Elastic hosiery, wigs and fabric supports Elastic support stockings are available on prescription, and are free to both men and women aged 60 or over. Support tights are available only through the hospital service but are free if you are entitled to free prescriptions; for example, if you receive Pension Credit Guarantee Credit or Pension Credit Guarantee Credit with Savings Credit or have certificate HC2.

Wigs and fabric supports are supplied through hospitals and are free for inpatients. If you are an outpatient, there are charges depending on the type of wig or fabric support supplied. However, they are free for you, your partner and any dependent young person under 20 if you receive Pension Credit Guarantee Credit or Pension Credit Guarantee Credit with Savings Credit or have certificate HC2; if you have certificate HC3, you may get some help with the cost.

Travel costs to receive NHS treatment If you get Pension Credit Guarantee Credit or Pension Credit Guarantee Credit with Savings Credit, you, your partner and any dependent young person under 20 are entitled to help with the necessary costs of travelling to hospital or other NHS premises to receive treatment arising from a referral by a doctor, dentist or consultant. You will need to ask the referring doctor or dentist whether the referral being made qualifies for help with travel costs. If parking charges are involved, these are included too.

If you have certificate HC2 or HC3 on grounds of low income, you may also get help towards these costs. (See page 178 on how to apply for a certificate.) If you are not sure what help you can get, speak to the doctor or dentist or contact the hospital before you travel. Hospitals will not normally reimburse taxi fares unless taxis are the only transport available – check with the hospital first.

If you qualify for help with travel costs and it is medically necessary for you to have a companion to accompany you, their travel costs should also be covered. However, they can be claimed only when they are certified to be necessary in the opinion of a doctor or appropriate health professional – so check with the doctor or hospital before you travel to ensure that you have the necessary permission or written confirmation.

There is no government scheme to help with costs of travelling to hospital to visit relatives or friends in hospital. However, if you are visiting a close relative in hospital and you receive Pension Credit (Guarantee Credit and/or Savings Credit), you may be able to get help with the cost of your fares from the Social Fund (see pages 90–95).

Healthcare outside the UK

As a UK resident, you are covered by the NHS only while you are in the UK. If you fall ill while abroad on business or on holiday, you may have to pay all or part of the cost of any treatment. There are special arrangements with member states of the EEA plus Switzerland (see pages vi–vii), which may entitle you to free or reduced-cost state-provided emergency treatment.

If you are in one of these countries, you must show your credit-card-sized plastic EHIC (European Health Insurance Card) to the doctor working for the state health system.

There is no charge for issuing an EHIC and you can apply for an EHIC by:

- calling the EHIC Application Line on 0845 606 2030. Your card will be delivered within 10 working days;
- completing an application form online (at www.ehic.org.uk); your card will be delivered within seven working days; or
- picking up an application form from a post office and returning your completed form to the address indicated; your card will be delivered within 21 working days.

You will need to have your NHS number or National Insurance number to hand when you apply.

The EHIC replaced the paper E111 and was introduced in January 2006. **EHICs issued early in 2006 are starting to expire. Always check the expiry date of your card well before you plan to travel, so that you have time to apply for a new EHIC.**

FOR MORE INFORMATION about an EHIC, or if you lose your EHIC, contact the EHIC enquiry line on 0845 605 0707.

The EHIC is not a substitute for holiday insurance and will only provide you with basic medical care in the event of an emergency. Not all doctors practising in an EEA country will be working within the state health system. So if you have to visit a doctor for emergency treatment, you may want to check whether your EHIC is acceptable to secure treatment and necessary medication is free of charge or at a reduced cost. You will also need to check that any hospital you visit for emergency treatment is part of the state health system.

It is advisable to take out private medical insurance to cover the full cost of any treatment you may need abroad, whether you are going to an EEA or non-EEA country.

When taking out insurance it is important that you declare pre-existing conditions you currently have or have had in the past, such as a heart attack. If you don't, you may not be covered by your policy should you make a claim. Medical treatment is very expensive, as is the cost of bringing a person back to the UK in the event of illness or death.

> FOR MORE INFORMATION, go to the Travel Abroad section of the NHS Choices website (www.nhs.uk). This contains information about non-EEA countries that the UK has reciprocal medical care agreements with and what you may be entitled to if you are taken ill in an EEA country. It also gives general guidance on immunisation requirements for travellers.

You are entitled to typhoid, polio and hepatitis A vaccines on the NHS: their administration is free and prescription charges follow your normal entitlement (free for people aged 60 and over, for example). All other travel immunisations are non-NHS and are likely to incur a variable charge.

If you are going to live permanently or for a large part of the year in another country, find out well in advance about your entitlement to medical treatment there. If you plan to return to the UK for holidays or for longer periods of time, you should also check your entitlement to treatment while you are back in the UK. Legislation passed in 2004 allows people in receipt of a UK State Pension who spend at least six months of the year living in the UK –

living the remainder of the year in an EEA country (as long as they are not registered as resident in that EEA country) – to be exempt from charges for NHS hospital treatment they receive while in the UK. This exemption does not apply if time outside the UK is spent in a non-EEA country.

If you live in another European Union (EU) member state and the UK covers the cost of your healthcare, new EU regulations mean that the UK, rather than the EU state where you live, may be responsible for issuing your EHIC from 1 May 2010. This would be the case if you receive your State Pension or other long-term benefit from the UK and you have registered the form E121 with the health authorities in the member state where you live. If this applies to you, you should have received a letter explaining this change along with an application form. If you have not been notified or need further information call the DWP Overseas Healthcare Team on 0191 218 1999. Your EHIC covers you when you travel from the EEA member state you live in to another EEA member country.

Bus services

In England older people and people with disabilities are entitled to a free bus pass and a minimum concession of free off-peak travel on buses in every area of the country, whether using the bus locally or when visiting other parts of the country.

It was announced in the Pre-Budget Report in December 2009 that the Government would re-establish the link between the age of eligibility for concessionary travel in England and the pensionable age. These changes took effect from 6 April 2010.

The age at which you are eligible for travel concessions for both men and women will rise in line with the incremental changes to State Pension age. Therefore, from 6 April 2010, the age of eligibility for travel concessions will be State Pension age for women and the pensionable age of a woman born on the same day for men.

With incremental changes, for example, a person who reaches age 60 on 6 April 2010 would be eligible for a concessionary bus pass on 6 May 2010. A person who reaches age 60 on 6 May 2010 would become eligible on 6 July 2010. The changes to the age of eligibility will not affect anyone already in possession of a bus pass. The changes will only affect those due to turn 60 on or after 6 April 2010.

See Chapter 1 for an explanation of the changes to State Pension age and the link to a calculator that enables people affected by the pension age changes to see at what age they become eligible for their State Pension and associated benefits.

Local authorities may also offer discounted travel on other modes of transport, such as trams or rail, at their discretion. Where local authorities offer more generous schemes, they can make a charge, as long as a free pass providing the statutory minimum remains available as an option.

In Wales and Scotland people over 60 and people with disabilities are entitled to free bus travel throughout the country.

FOR MORE INFORMATION, contact your local authority (district or unitary council), or, in metropolitan areas, the Passenger Transport Executive (PTE).

Coach services

People who are aged 60 and over, and people who have a local authority concessionary travel pass because they are disabled, may be able to get coach fares at half price in

England and Wales. Participation in this scheme is voluntary but National Express, the major provider, is part of the scheme. The offer might not be available during some peak periods or on some tickets.

In Scotland the same rules apply as for bus concessions.

Rail and underground

All rail companies give one-third reductions on most types of ticket to people who have a Senior Railcard, which currently costs £26 and is valid for one year, or £65 for three years. It is available to people aged 60 or over, provided proof of age is given.

Leaflets with application forms should be available from any staffed railway stations or rail-appointed travel agents or from the website www.senior-railcard.co.uk.

If you are disabled, you can buy a Disabled Person's Railcard, which currently costs £18 for one year or £48 for three years, and which allows you and a companion to travel at a third off most standard fares.

APPLICATION FORMS AND FULL DETAILS OF WHO QUALIFIES are available from many railway stations or from the Disabled Persons Railcard Office at the address on page 207 or the website (www.disabledpersons-railcard.co.uk).

People travelling in their own wheelchair who do not hold the Railcard can get discounts on single and return tickets. They can get the same discounts for one travelling companion. Registered blind and partially sighted people without a Railcard can also get discounts, but only if they travel with a companion.

Underground or other transport systems may also offer concessions; ask at local offices.

In Northern Ireland the concessionary travel scheme is called Smartpass and it provides free public transport on scheduled bus and rail services throughout Northern Ireland to men and women aged 60 or over or those registered blind and war disablement pensioners. The Smartpass also enables free travel in the Republic of Ireland to those aged 65 and over. You can pick up an application form at any bus station, or by telephoning 0845 600 0049.

Taxicard schemes

Some local authorities operate taxicard schemes, which provide reduced fares for disabled people. Contact your local authority to find out if it runs a scheme.

Airlines

Some airlines may have concessionary fares for pensioners. Ask at the airline or travel agent for details.

FOR MORE INFORMATION about concessions on public transport see Age UK Factsheet 26 Public Transport and Concessions. *Also, for details about help with the costs of travel, contact Age UK Advice on 0800 169 65 65. Callers in Scotland can contact the Scottish Helpline for Older People (SHOP) on 0845 125 9732.*

OTHER CONCESSIONS

People over a certain age or who are entitled to a State Pension may be able to receive concessions such as: reductions at leisure centres and swimming pools; lower admission prices to places of interest; and sometimes reduced fees for joining adult education classes. Most national museums now have free entry. Sometimes local businesses such as hairdressers may have special rates at certain times of the week. These concessions vary, so look out for any reductions that might apply to you.

Television

Television licences are free for households with a person aged 75 and over.

There are two other types of concession. People who are registered blind can obtain a 50% reduction from the full licence fee. It is also possible to get specially adapted TV sound receivers and these do not need a licence to operate. Some people over the State Pension age who live in care homes or certain sheltered accommodation qualify for a concessionary £7.50 licence.

FOR MORE INFORMATION see Age UK Factsheet 3 Television Licence Concessions, *or contact TV Licensing on 0844 800 6790 or go to their website (www.tvlicensing.co.uk).*

Digital Switchover Help Scheme   The digital switchover will be taking place between 2008 and 2012, ITV region by ITV region. This means that, once the transition is completed in your region, you will need to have digital equipment to continue watching television. Some people will receive support with installation and use of digital TV equipment.

The Help Scheme is available to people who are aged 75 or over, or registered blind or partially sighted, or entitled to DLA or AA (or equivalent). Help will be free for those who are eligible and who also receive Income Support, income-based JSA, income-related ESA or Pension Credit; other eligible people will have to pay a subsidised one-off fee of £40.

If you are eligible for help, you will be sent details of the scheme before your area goes digital and you will need to respond to the letter.

FOR MORE INFORMATION, call Age UK Advice on 0800 169 65 65. Callers in Scotland can contact the Scottish Helpline for Older People (SHOP) on 0845 125 9732.

More information is also available from the Digital UK website (www.digitaluk.co.uk) or phone them on 0845 6505050 (local rate).

Passports

Since 18 October 2004, British citizens born on or before 2 September 1929 have been eligible for free 10-year passports. These are renewable on expiry without charge. Those who are eligible and purchased a passport between 19 May 2004 and 18 October 2004 are able to apply for a refund by writing to their regional passport office.

FOR MORE INFORMATION, go to the Identity and Passport Service website (www.ips.gov.uk) or contact the Passport Adviceline on 0300 222 0000.

HELP FROM CHARITIES AND BENEVOLENT FUNDS

If you have checked that you are getting all the benefits you are entitled to and it is still hard to manage financially, you could try asking for help from charities or benevolent funds. Assistance may be available either as a lump sum or regular weekly payments. If you are receiving Pension Credit (see pages 46–70), all charitable payments made to you will be ignored.

Benevolent funds help people in particular circumstances – for example, these might be based on your occupation (or former occupation) or that of your partner; any health problems or disabilities you may have; or the area where you live. Others may help people who are members of trade unions or who have a particular religious belief.

FOR MORE INFORMATION, contact a local advice agency. There are also two national organisations – The Association of Charity Officers and Charity Search – that can help put people in contact with charities and benevolent funds. Their addresses are on pages 205 and 206.

LEGAL FEES, WILLS AND FUNERALS

Help with legal costs and making wills

If you need help with a legal problem, you may be able to obtain this free from a local advice agency or you may be eligible for Legal Aid to help with the costs of a solicitor's fees. If you are on Pension Credit, income-related ESA, Income Support or income-based JSA, or have a low income and little or no savings, you may be able to obtain help with legal advice and representation through the different Legal Aid schemes. This can include help with solicitors' fees for making a will, but in England and Wales you must be 70 or over or mentally or physically disabled in order to receive help. Community Legal Advice, run by the Legal Services Commission, can advise you whether you qualify for Legal Aid, and can provide free legal advice on some subjects if you qualify.

FOR MORE INFORMATION, contact Age UK Advice on 0800 169 65 65 or Community Legal Advice on 0845 345 4345 or through their website (www.communitylegaladvice.org.uk). The Scottish Legal Aid Board also publishes leaflets on Legal Aid. Its address is on page 210.

Help with funeral payments

This section describes the Funeral Payments, available from the Social Fund, which are part of the social security system. For more details about arranging a funeral, including information about the duty of local and health authorities to pay for certain funerals, contact Age UK Advice on 0800 169 65 65.

You may be able to receive a Social Fund Funeral Payment towards the cost of a funeral if you have good reason for taking responsibility for the expenses and you or your partner are receiving Pension Credit, Income Support,

Housing Benefit, Council Tax Benefit, income-based JSA, income-related ESA, Child Tax Credit at a rate higher than the family element or Working Tax Credit where a disability or severe disability element is included in the award. Any savings you have will not be taken into account. However, as explained below, there are restrictions on who can receive a payment and limits on the amount of the payment, so it is very important to check what you are entitled to before making the arrangements.

To receive a payment you should be the partner of the person who has died, or someone else who it is reasonable to expect to take responsibility for arranging the funeral. The person who died must have been ordinarily resident in the UK and the funeral must normally take place in the UK, but in some circumstances it can take place elsewhere in a Member State of the EU, Iceland, Liechtenstein, Norway or Switzerland.

Unless you are the partner of the person who has died, the decision-maker may decide, based on the nature and extent of your contact with the person who has died, that it was not reasonable for you to have taken responsibility for the funeral costs. The payment can cover necessary burial and cremation costs, certain necessary travel expenses and up to £700 for other funeral expenses. If there is a pre-paid funeral plan, the Social Fund payment cannot help with items covered by the plan. If the pre-paid plan does not cover expenses such as the cost of a coffin, any religious costs, flowers, other transport costs, etc., then the payment could be up to £120.

If money is available from the estate of the person who has died, or from insurance policies or pre-paid funeral plans, this will be deducted from any award that would otherwise be made.

To make a claim you will need form SF200 from Jobcentre Plus. You have to claim within three months of the funeral, but it is advisable to talk to someone from your local Jobcentre Plus office to check what you are entitled to before arranging a funeral.

FOR MORE INFORMATION, contact Jobcentre Plus – their number is in the business section of your phone book – or contact Age UK Advice on 0800 169 65 65 to order the information guide When Someone Dies *or see DWP leaflet D49* What to Do after a Death.

Further Information

This part of *Your Rights to Money Benefits* gives details about local and national sources of assistance and advice plus information about getting hold of Department for Work and Pensions (DWP) leaflets, Age UK information, and the other publications on benefits mentioned in the book. It also includes an index to help you find the information you need plus a summary of the main benefit rates.

DEPARTMENT FOR WORK AND PENSIONS

Much of the information in *Your Rights to Money Benefits* covers State Pensions and benefits. The government department responsible is the DWP. The rules for State Pensions and benefits and the levels of payment are set out in legislation – for example, each year regulations are agreed in Parliament, setting out the annual increases to pensions and benefits.

In April 2008, The Pension Service and the Disability and Carers Service were brought together as a single agency – the Pension, Disability and Carers Service. In the short term, however, as far as customers are concerned the services will continue to operate as before, with the same names and numbers, so they are described separately below and throughout this book.

The Pension Service is the part of the DWP responsible for State Pensions, Pension Credit and Winter Fuel Payments, and for providing information about other pension-related entitlements, including State Pension forecasts to help those of working age in planning for their future.

The Disability and Carers Service is responsible for Attendance Allowance, Disability Living Allowance and Carer's Allowance.

Jobcentre Plus deals with people of working age by administering benefits and providing advice and support about employment opportunities. It is also responsible for Social Fund payments (other than Winter Fuel Payments). Details of your local Jobcentre Plus office can be found in the phone book.

Problems with administration

If you have a problem with the administration of a benefit – for example, if there is a delay in processing your claim – you can complain to The Pension Service by phone, letter or email, or by using leaflet GL22 *Tell Us How to Improve our Service*. If you are still dissatisfied, get in touch with a local advice agency or your MP.

The Pension Service

The Pension Service delivers services and products through a network of pension centres across England, Scotland and Wales. The pension centres deal with customers by phone, post or email, and are supported by a local service that offers face-to-face contact. There is also a National Pension Centre and phone lines covering specific aspects of State Pensions and benefits.

To contact The Pension Service, phone 0845 606 0265 (8.00am–8.00pm weekdays; textphone 0845 606 0285) – this will connect you with the pension centre covering your area. Welsh language customers living in Wales phone 0845 606 0275 (textphone 0845 606 0295). Staff there will provide information and answer queries about your State Pension and other pension-related entitlements. They can also tell you about local services, including details of information points in your area and home visits. You can find the postal or email address of your pension centre on the Direct Gov website (www.direct.gov.uk).

National/International Pension Service addresses and phone lines You are encouraged to use the phone to contact The Pension Service, but if you prefer to write, you can use the following address for The National Pension Centre and the International Pension Centre: The Pension Service, Tyneview Park, Whitley Road, Benton, Newcastle upon Tyne NE98 1BA.

State Pension Forecasting Service

For a State Pension forecast, phone 0845 300 0168 (textphone 0845 300 0169). Forecasts can be obtained up to 30 days prior to reaching State Pension age (see page 3).

Call the Future Pension Centre (0845 300 0168) and they
will help you to fill in the form; lines are open from 8.00am
to 8.00pm Monday to Friday and 9.00am to 1.00pm on
Saturday. If you have hearing or speech difficulties and
have a textphone, call textphone 0845 300 0169.
Alternatively, write to State Pension Forecasting, Tyneview
Park, Whitley Road, Benton, Newcastle upon Tyne NE98 1BA
and ask for a forecast application form (BR19) and a return
envelope. It will take an average of 12 working days to
prepare your forecast from the date your application form is
received. The forecast application form is available in
English and Welsh. If you do not speak English or Welsh, an
interpreter can be arranged.

Pensions Direct

Deals with changes of circumstances and enquiries for
people who have their pension paid direct into an account.
Tel: 0845 301 3011, 8.00am–8.00pm weekdays. Textphone:
0845 301 3012.

International Pension Centre

For information about pensions and medical cover for
those who live, or have previously lived, overseas. Tel: 0191
218 7777, 8.00am–8.00pm weekdays. Textphone: 0191
218 7280. International Pension Centre, Tyneview Park,
Newcastle Upon Tyne NE98 1BA.

Pension Credit

To apply for Pension Credit by phone, or to get an
application form, phone 0800 99 1234 (free call),
8.00am–8.00pm weekdays, 9.00am–1.00pm Saturdays.
Textphone: 0800 169 0133.

Disability and Carers Service

Disability Contact and Processing Unit, Warbreck House,
Warbreck Hill, Blackpool FY2 0YE.

Tel: 0845 7123456, 7.30am–6.30pm weekdays. Textphone: 0845 7224433 (you can also use the RNID Typetalk service).

The Pension, Disability and Carers Service administers Disability Living Allowance and Attendance Allowance, although initial claims are normally dealt with at the regionally based Disability Benefit Centres.

Carer's Allowance Unit, Palatine House, Lancaster Road, Preston, Lancashire PR1 1HB.

Tel: 0845 608 4321, 9am–5.00pm Mondays–Thursdays, 9am–4.30pm Fridays. Textphone: 0845 604 5312.

Benefit Enquiry Line for people with disabilities and carers. Advice and information for disabled people and carers on the range of benefits available.

Tel: 0800 88 22 00 (a free call), 8.30am–6.30pm weekdays, 9.00am–1.00pm Saturdays. Textphone: 0800 24 33 55 (you can also use the RNID Typetalk service).

Staff can arrange for help with completing forms over the phone for benefits such as Attendance Allowance and Disability Living Allowance.

DWP/Pension Service websites

If you have access to the internet, you can get leaflets, publications and other information from the websites. You can also download claim forms for many benefits. Websites: www.dwp.gov.uk, www.thepensionservice.gov.uk and www.direct.gov.uk

AGE UK ADVICE

Age UK Advice is a service for older people, their relatives and friends and those who care for and work with them. Our advice line provides free written information on a wide range of subjects affecting older people, including money and benefits, finding and paying for care, housing issues, health services and healthy living, consumer issues, common legal questions for older people and age discrimination and employment.

We can be contacted by calling 0800 169 65 65 (8am–7pm, 7 days a week) or by writing to: Age UK, Freepost (SWB 30375), Ashburton, Devon TQ13 7ZZ. All of Age UK's range of information can also be viewed and downloaded free from our website (www.ageuk.org.uk).

Materials available include information guides that introduce subjects, and detailed factsheets for professionals and individuals who have a specific enquiry or problem. To receive a free email update when new and updated Age UK information products are published, fill in your details at www.ageuk.org.uk/infoupdate

Where possible, Age UK's information is applicable across the UK. There are differences in the law between England, Northern Ireland, Scotland and Wales, however, so for some subjects enquirers from these nations may be provided with different versions of materials or signposted to their national office.

Callers in Scotland can contact the Scottish Helpline for Older People (SHOP) on 0845 125 9732, 10am–4pm weekdays, run by Age UK in Scotland.

LOCAL SOURCES OF HELP

Age UK/Age Concern*
Most areas have a local Age UK/Age Concern* that provides services and advice. You can find the address from the phone book, library or Citizens Advice, or you can write to

*Many local Age Concerns are changing their name to Age UK.

the appropriate national office in Wales, Scotland or Northern Ireland (addresses on page 224) or call Age UK Advice (0800 169 65 65) for the address of the local Age UK/Age Concern* nearest to you.

Citizens Advice

The local offices provide advice and information on all kinds of subjects, including benefits, housing and consumer problems. You can find out where your nearest Citizens Advice is from the phone book or at your local library. The Citizens Advice website (www.adviceguide.org.uk) offers advice on a range of issues such as employment, consumer advice and benefits.

Law centre

There may be a law centre giving free legal advice in your area. Check in the phone book or at a Citizens Advice, or contact Community Legal Advice, Tel: 0845 345 4345. Community Legal Advice (which is funded by the Legal Services Commission) also offers information about your rights and how to obtain legal advice, and its website (www.communitylegaladvice.org.uk) gives useful legal information. The Law Centres Federation website (www.lawcentres.org.uk) may also be of interest.

Local authority/council

In England, the structure of local government depends on whether you live in a county, or in a metropolitan or London borough, or a unitary authority. All areas in Scotland and Wales have a unitary authority. In England, if you live in a county, the district council will deal with Housing Benefit, Council Tax Benefit and other matters to do with the Council Tax. You will need to contact the county council about social services. In a metropolitan or

*Many local Age Concerns are changing their name to Age UK.

London borough, or unitary authority, there will be just one authority that will deal with the Council Tax, Housing Benefit and social services. Some authorities have welfare rights workers to advise on benefits. You will find the address of your local authority in the phone book under the name of your county, unitary authority, metropolitan or London borough, or ask at your local library.

Local councillor

A councillor for your area may be able to help with problems with the local authority. You can get the names of the councillors for your 'ward' from the town hall, library or Citizens Advice.

Local Government Ombudsman

If you feel you have suffered because of maladministration in the way the local authority has dealt with your case, you can make a complaint to the Local Government Ombudsman (or the Scottish Public Services Ombudsman or the Public Services Ombudsman for Wales). You can do this direct or through your local councillor. Ask a local advice agency or councillor for further information or look at the website at www.lgo.org.uk – www.spso.org.uk in Scotland or www.ombudsman-wales.org.uk in Wales.

Member of Parliament (MP)

Your MP may be able to help with problems involving government departments. If you do not know who your MP is, ask at the town hall, library or Citizens Advice or ring the House of Commons Information Office, Tel: 020 7219 4272. Most MPs hold regular surgeries locally; or you can write to your MP at the House of Commons, London SW1A 0AA. For a complaint about unfair treatment by a government department (for example, a delay with a benefit claim), ask the MP to refer your complaint to the Parliamentary Ombudsman.

In Scotland you can contact Members of the Scottish Parliament at Scottish Parliament, Edinburgh EH99 1SP or Tel: 0131 348 5000.

In Wales you can contact Assembly Members at the National Assembly for Wales, Cardiff Bay, Cardiff CF99 1NA or ring the Public Information and Education Team Tel: 0845 010 5500 (local rate).

Trade union

If you were a member of a trade union before retirement, it may be worth contacting your local branch, particularly for problems over a pension from work.

Welfare rights and money advice centres

There may be an independent welfare rights or money advice centre locally. Money advice centres generally deal with debt problems and may only accept referrals from other agencies.

NATIONAL SOURCES OF INFORMATION

The national organisations listed below may be able to help or put you in touch with a source of advice.

Association of Charity Officers

Five Ways, 57–59 Hatfield Road, Potters Bar, Hertfordshire EN6 1HS.
Tel: 01707 651 777, weekdays 10.00am–4.00pm
www.aco.uk.net
Provides information about charities that make grants to individuals in need.

Care and Repair Forum Scotland

135 Buchanan St, Suite 2.5, Glasgow G1 2JA.
Tel: 0141 221 9879
www.careandrepairscotland.co.uk
The national co-ordinating body for Home Improvement Agencies in Scotland.

Carers UK

20 Great Dover Street, London SE1 4LX.
Tel: 020 7378 4999
CarersLine: 0808 808 7777, Wednesdays–Thursdays
10.00am–12.00pm and 2.00pm–4.00pm
www.carersuk.org
Provides general advice and help for all carers.

Charity Search

Freepost (BS 6610), Avonmouth, Bristol BS11 9TW.
Tel: 0117 982 4060, Mondays–Thursdays 9.30am–2.30pm
www.charitysearch.org.uk
Helps link older people with charities that may provide grants to individuals. Applications in writing are preferred.

Counsel and Care

Twyman House, 16 Bonny Street, London NW1 9PG.
Tel: 0845 300 7585 (advice line), weekdays
10.00am–4.00pm, except Wednesdays 10.00am–1.00pm
www.counselandcare.org.uk
Advises on obtaining and paying for care in a care home and a range of community care issues.

Disability Alliance

Universal House, 88–94 Wentworth Street, London E1 7SA.
Tel: 020 7247 8776
www.disabilityalliance.org
Produces the Disability Rights Handbook *and other publications, and gives advice on social security benefits for disabled people.*

Disabled Persons Railcard Office
Rail Travel Made Easy, PO Box 11631, Laurencekirk
AB30 9AA.
Tel: 0845 605 0525 (application helpline)
Textphone: 0845 601 0132
www.disabledpersons-railcard.co.uk
For a railcard offering concessionary fares.

EAGA Partnership Ltd
Freephone 0800 316 2808 (England)
Freephone 0800 316 2815 (Wales)
www.eaga.co.uk
Administers the Warm Front grants in England and Home Energy Efficiency Scheme in Wales.

Energy Saving Scotland Advice Centre (ESSAC)
Energy Saving Trust
2nd Floor, Ocean Point 1, 94 Ocean Drive, Edinburgh EH6 6JH
Tel: 0800 512 012
www.energysavingtrust.org.uk/scotland
Administers the Energy Assistance Package throughout Scotland.

Foundations
Bleaklow House, Howard Town Mill, Glossop SK13 8HT.
Tel: 01457 891909
www.foundations.uk.com
The national co-ordinating body for Home Improvement Agencies in England.

HM Revenue & Customs National Insurance Contributions Office (NICO)
Benton Park View, Newcastle upon Tyne NE98 1ZZ.
Tel: 0845 302 1479
www.hmrc.gov.uk/nic
For information about NI contributions and records and Statutory Sick Pay (SSP). HM Revenue & Customs (formerly the Inland Revenue) is also responsible for tax credits. To find details of offices and HMRC Tax Enquiry Centres, look in

the phone book under 'Inland Revenue' or 'HM Revenue & Customs'.

If your employer does not pay you SSP, or pays you less than you think they should, ask them to give you the reason in writing. If you disagree with their reason, you can contact HM Revenue & Customs Employees Enquiry Line on 0845 302 1479.

Home Energy Efficiency Scheme

Tel: 0800 316 2815

www.heeswales.co.uk

Home Energy Efficiency Schemes are available in Wales. Also, see Warm Front for people living in England and Energy Assistance Package for people living in Scotland.

Independent Living Fund

PO Box 7525, Nottingham NG2 4ZT.

Tel: 0845 601 8815 / 0115 945 0700

www.ilf.org.uk

For information and a user guide about the ILF.

Motability

City Gate House, 22 Southwark Bridge Road, London SE1 9HB.

Tel: 0845 456 4566

www.motability.co.uk

The Motability Scheme offers help to people in receipt of either the higher rate of the mobility component of Disability Living Allowance or the War Pensioners' Mobility Supplement. Offers the chance to buy or lease a car at an affordable price. May also be able to offer financial help towards the cost of a suitable car, adaptations, driving lessons or a wheelchair-accessible vehicle.

Passenger Transport Executive (PTE)

Wellington House, 40-50 Wellington Street, LEEDS LS1 2DE.
Tel: (0113) 251 7204
Fax: (0113) 251 7333
The six PTEs provide, plan, procure and promote public transport in six of England's largest conurbations: Greater Manchester, Merseyside, South Yorkshire, Tyne and Wear, West Midlands and West Yorkshire.

The Pensions Advisory Service (TPAS)

11 Belgrave Road, London SW1V 1RB.
Tel: 0845 601 2923 (pensions helpline)
Tel: 0845 600 0806 (women & pensions helpline)
www.opas.org.uk
Offers help and advice about pensions. Will also help anyone with a problem with their occupational or personal pension arrangement.

Royal National Institute of Blind People (RNIB)

105 Judd Street, London WC1H 9NE.
Tel: 020 7388 1266
Tel: 0303 123 9999 (helpline)
www.rnib.org.uk
Offers advice and information on social security and other issues for blind and partially sighted people.

Royal National Institute for Deaf People (RNID)

RNID Information Line, 19–23 Featherstone Street, London EC1Y 8SL.
Tel: 020 7296 8000
Tel: 0808 808 0123 (freephone helpline)
Tel: 0808 808 9000 (freephone textphone)
www.rnid.org.uk
Provides information for deaf and hard-of-hearing people.

Scottish Legal Aid Board (SLAB)
44 Drumsheugh Gardens, Edinburgh EH3 7SW.
Tel: 0131 226 7061
Tel: 0845 122 8686 (legal aid helpline)
www.slab.org.uk
Publishes leaflets about Legal Aid for people in Scotland.

Service Personnel and Veterans Agency
Norcross, Thornton Cleveleys, Lancashire FY5 3WP.
Tel: 0800 169 2277 (helpline), Mondays–Thursdays
8.15am–5.15pm, Fridays 8.15am–4.30pm
Tel: 0800 169 3458 (textphone)
www.veterans-uk.info
Responsible for the War Pensions Scheme and is also the point of contact within the Ministry of Defence for information and advice on issues of concern to veterans and their families.

Warm Front
Customer Response Team, Eaga House, Archbold Terrace, Jesmond, Newcastle Upon Tyne NE2 1DB.
Tel: 0800 316 2805
Tel: 0800 316 6011 (customer service)
www.warmfront.co.uk
Warm Front grants are available in England. Also, see Home Energy Efficiency Scheme for people living in Wales and Energy Assistance Package for people living in Scotland.

> *FOR MORE INFORMATION about national organisations in Scotland, Wales and Northern Ireland, contact the appropriate national Age UK (addresses on page 224).*

FURTHER READING

Government leaflets As well as the leaflets mentioned in *Your Rights to Money Benefits*, there is a catalogue of all the DWP leaflets produced (Cat1) on the DWP website (www.dwp.gov.uk). The leaflets should be available from your local Jobcentre Plus office or pension centre, and they are sometimes in libraries, post offices or Citizens Advice offices or www.direct.gov.uk. Most of the information formerly available from The Pension Service website has been moved to the Direct Gov website.

HM Revenue & Customs (formerly the Inland Revenue) deals with issues relating to NI contributions. Leaflets on contributions can be obtained from tax offices or on the HMRC website (www.hmrc.gov.uk).

Leaflets about help with health costs are available from the NHS Forms Orderline.
Tel: 0845 610 1112
www.dh.gov.uk/helpwithhealthcosts
There is also a health cost advice line. Tel: 0845 850 1166.

Other publications

For detailed information on services and benefits for disabled people, you may wish to get the *Disability Rights Handbook*, available from the Disability Alliance, Universal House, 88–94 Wentworth Street, London E1 7SA. Tel: 020 7247 8776 or www.disabilityalliance.org.

For detailed information on all benefits, with reference to the relevant government legislation, you may wish to refer to the *Welfare Benefits and Tax Credits Handbook 2010/11*, £39 plus post and packing (£9.00 post free for individual benefit claimants), which is available from the Child Poverty Action Group (CPAG), 94 White Lion Street, London N1 9PF. Tel: 020 7837 7979; website: www.cpag.org.uk. This book covers both means-tested and non-means-tested benefits.

These books may also be available for reference at your local library.

BENEFIT RATES APRIL 2010/11

Some of the main weekly benefit rates are listed below for quick reference:

State Pensions and disability benefits

Attendance Allowance

higher rate	£71.40
lower rate	£47.80

Disability Living Allowance
Care component

highest rate	£71.40
middle rate	£47.80
lowest rate	£18.95

Mobility component

higher rate	£49.85
lower rate	£18.95

Carer's Allowance £53.90

Incapacity Benefit (long-term rate) £91.40

Severe Disablement Allowance (basic rate) £59.45

Basic State Pension

basic rate	£97.65
wife on husband's contributions	£58.50
couple on husband's contributions	£156.15

Income-related benefits

Housing Benefit/Council Tax Benefit standard applicable amounts for people aged 65 or over

single person	£153.15
couple	£229.50

**Pension Credit standard appropriate amounts and
Housing Benefit/Council Tax Benefit standard applicable
amounts for people of Pension Credit qualifying age but
under 65 (see page 46)**

single person	£132.60
couple	£202.40

Pension Credit maximum savings credit

single person	£20.52
couple	£27.09

Premiums/additions

Severe disability

single	£53.65
couple (one qualifies)	£53.65
couple (both qualify)	£107.30
carer	£30.05

KEEPING UP TO DATE

This edition of *Your Rights to Money Benefits* is based on
the information available in April 2010. The benefit levels
will normally apply until the first week in April 2011. A new
edition of the book will be published next year to cover the
period from April 2011 to April 2012. However, sometimes
changes are made during the course of a year.

If you would like us to inform you of any major changes introduced before April 2011, please photocopy or cut off this page and return it to the address below.

Write in with your details if you do not want to cut up the book.

Dear Age UK

Please send me details about any major changes introduced before April 2011

Name (block letters)

_____

Signature

_____

Address

_____

_____

_____

_____

Postcode

_____

Please return to:
Age UK (YR Update)
FREEPOST (SWB 30375)
Ashburton
Devon TQ13 7ZZ

INDEX

State Pension *see* Additional
State Pension; Basic State
Pension; Graduated
Retirement Benefit; State
Second Pension (S2P)
State Pension Forecasting
Service 199–200
State Second Pension (S2P)
23–27
Carer Credits 24
contracting out 24–26
Statutory Sick Pay (SSP) 115
Supporting People fund 135

T
tax
Additional State Pension 22
impact from deferring your
State Pension 33
working after State Pension
age 37
taxicard schemes 190
telephone costs 162
television licences 191
terminal illness, and Disability
Benefits 108–109
The Pensions Advisory Service
(TPAS) 40
trade unions 205
travel costs, help with 184
airlines 190
bus services 187–188
coach services 188–189
passports 192
rail and underground travel
189–190
taxicard schemes 190
tribunals, benefits 43–44

U
unemployment
Jobseeker's Allowance (JSA)
14, 35, 151–154

V
Vulnerable Groups Scheme
(WaterSure) 161

W
war pensions 126
Warm Front grants 166–167
water charges 161
welfare rights 205
widows, widowers and surviving
civil partners
Additional State Pension
26–27
Graduated Retirement Benefit
28
State Pensions 5, 9–11
Widow's Pension 158–159
wigs 183
wills, making 193
Winter Fuel Payments 165
work *see* also personal pension
schemes
after State Pension age 36–37
and Employment and Support
Allowance (ESA) 115–120
Statutory Sick Pay (SSP) 115
Working Tax Credit 35, 150–151

Age UK
1268 London Road
London
SW16 4ER
Tel: 020 8765 7200
www.ageuk.org.uk

Age Cymru
Ty John Pathy
13 and 14 Neptune Court
Vanguard Way
Cardiff, CF24 5PJ
Tel: 029 2043 1555
www.agecymru.org.uk

Age Scotland
Causewayside House
160 Causewayside
Edinburgh, EH9 1PR
Tel: 0845 833 0200
www.agescotland.org.uk

Age NI
3 Lower Crescent
Belfast
BT7 1NR
Tel: 028 9024 5729
www.ageni.org

AGE UK BOOKS

Age UK publishes a wide range of bestselling books that help thousands of people each year. Our books provide practical, trusted advice on a range of subjects, from finance and retirement planning to health and surfing the web. Whether you are acting as a carer or want to know more about your rights to healthcare or employment, we have something for everyone.

To find out more, to order a free catalogue or to buy a book please call our hotline on 0870 44 22 120 or visit the website at www.ageuk.org.uk/bookshop. You can also buy our books from all good bookshops.

AGE UK INFORMATION GUIDES

Age UK produce a range of comprehensive information guides that answer many of the questions older people – or those advising them – may have. These free guides cover issues such as housing, care homes, pensions, benefits, health, community care, leisure and education, and can be obtained by calling Age UK Advice on 0800 169 65 65 or by downloading them from the website: www.ageuk.org.uk/publications.